Eat Healthier

Tips for healthy eating

Haytham Al Fiqi

ISBN: 1530270960

ISBN-13: 978-1530270965

1- Eat a variety of veggies for a healthier you

The new food guidelines issued by the United States government recommend that all Americans eat between five and nine servings of fruits and vegetables each and every day. When you first hear that number, it may seem like a lot, but it is actually much easier than you think to fit that many servings of fruits and vegetables into your daily diet. For one thing, the shelves of the grocery stores are fairly bursting with fresh fruits and vegetables. In addition, vegetables and fruits are some of the least expensive, most nutrient rich, foods in the supermarket. With all these fruits and vegetables to choose from, it is very easy to make these nutritious, delicious foods part of your daily meals and snacks.

When you take into account how much a serving really is, it is actually quite easy to get five to nine servings of fruits and vegetables per day. For instance, the recommended daily amount actually equates to a quite reasonable two cups of fruit and two and a half cups of vegetables every day. When you consider how many fruits and vegetables are available, and how low the prices usually are, it is easy to see how easy to reach this daily goal really is.

One great way to get the nutrients you need from fruits and vegetables every day is to take full advantage of the variety of these foods available. Eating the same thing every day quickly becomes boring, so why not pick a variety of fruits and vegetables, in every color of the rainbow and in every conceivable shape, size and texture, to give yourself a varied diet every day.

When shopping for fruits and vegetables, it is important to choose a variety of different colors. This is for more than purely artistic reasons. Different color fruits and vegetables have different types of nutrients, and choosing a variety of colors will help ensure you get all the vitamins and minerals you need each and every day.

Finding new recipes is another great way to ensure you get those five to nine servings of fruits and vegetables every day. Everyone likes to try out new recipes, and these new recipes may just provide the impetus you need to eat all those fruits and veggies.

New recipes can also provide you the important opportunity to, try out some fruits and vegetables you have never tried before. For instance, everyone has eaten oranges, but have you tried kiwi fruit or mangoes? How about spinach or kale? Trying new things is a great way to find new favorites while getting the best nutrition available.

Many people mistakenly think that they do not need to eat five to nine servings of fruits and vegetables every day if they just take a vitamin supplement. Actually, nothing could be further from the truth. That is because fruits and vegetables contain far more than the micronutrients identified by science and synthesized in vitamin pills. While these micronutrients, such as vitamin C, vitamin A and vitamin E are important to good health, so too are the hundreds of other elements that are contained in healthy foods like fruits and vegetables. These elements are not available in any pill, they must be ingested through a healthy, balanced diet that contains plenty of fruits and vegetables.

In addition, fruits and vegetables are much less costly than vitamin pills. Fruits and vegetables are very inexpensive, especially when purchased in season and grown locally. In the long run, getting the nutrition you need from the food you eat is much less expensive, and much better for you, than popping those vitamin pills every day.

So don't forget to get your five to nine servings of fruits and vegetables every day. It may seem like a lot, but you can meet this quite reasonable goal simply by including fruits and vegetables as snacks, as garnishes, as side dishes and as meals.

2- Eat a wide variety of foods for a healthy diet

One of the most frequently cited reasons that diets and attempts at healthy eating fail is boredom. Many people simply do not know how to keep a healthy diet interesting day after day, and it can be quite a challenge.

Given the huge variety of fruits, vegetables, whole grains, meats and other healthy foods at the local grocery store, however, it is definitely possible to create exciting, nutritious meals that will keep boredom at bay.

Your key to healthy eating

The key to the success of any plan for healthy eating is to eat what you like, but to exercise moderation when it comes to the less healthy foods. Improving your level of health and fitness does not mean forgoing that piece of chocolate cake, for instance. It does mean, however, limiting yourself to one piece. A healthy diet contains all types of foods, including carbohydrates, proteins, and even fats. The key is choosing foods that provide the best combination of taste and nutrition. After all, if your diet consists of foods you hate, you will not stick with it.

The revised USDA food pyramid contains five major food groups – grains, vegetables, fruits, milk and dairy, and meat and beans. When choosing foods from these groups, it is important to eat a wide variety of foods from every food group. Doing so will not only give you a great deal of variety and keep boredom from setting in, but it will provide the best nutritional balance as well. In addition the widely known micronutrients, such as vitamin A, vitamin D, vitamin C, etc. all foods contain a variety of macronutrients, like fats, proteins, fiber and water. Though present in extremely tiny amounts, micronutrients are vitally important to good health. That is why a healthy, varied diet is so important.

In addition, when choosing foods from within the various food groups, some choices are naturally better and healthier than others. For instance, choosing skim or 2% milk instead of full fat whole milk is a good way to cut down on both fat and calories. And choosing poultry or lean meat is a great way to get the protein you need every day without extra fat, cholesterol and calories.

Likewise cereals and breads that carry the whole grain label are healthier than those who do not. Even in the world of fruits and vegetables some choices are better than others. For instance, peaches packed in heavy syrup add unnecessary sugar to the diet, while those packed in water or juice provide only good nutrition.

There has been a trend lately to add vitamin fortification to food, and this can sometimes be a good way to maximize nutrition. It is important to remember, however, that proper nutrition comes from a healthy diet, not from vitamin supplements. It is fine to buy calcium fortified cereal, but the bulk of your calcium intake should still come from milk, dairy products and green leafy veggies.

Choosing the best foods

Knowing the five major food groups and how much of each to eat every day is only part of the picture. The other part is choosing the best foods from within those food groups. That means things like choosing the leanest cuts of meat, using egg substitutes instead of whole eggs, choosing the freshest fruits and vegetables, etc.

Even with fruits and vegetables, some choices are better than others. Some fruits, such as avocados, for instance, are packed with fat and calories. It is important to check the nutritional qualities of the fruits and vegetables you buy, and not simply assume that all fruits and vegetables are equally healthy.

One way to maximize nutrition while minimizing cost is to buy fruits and vegetables that are in season. Fruits and vegetables that are in season are usually quite a bit cheaper than those that must be shipped hundreds or even thousands of miles, and they are generally much fresher too. Of course, depending on where you live, there may be varieties of fruits and vegetables that are not available locally, so the northerner in search of citrus fruits will just have to watch the sales and buy accordingly.

3- Understanding fats and carbs

Fats and carbohydrates are two building blocks of a healthy diet, but many people do not understand their role in proper nutrition. While the daily intake of fats and oils should be limited, these elements are still a vital part of the diet. The key is to make smart choices when it comes to fats and oils. That means substituting saturated fats with unsaturated fats, and using healthier, lighter oils in cooking.

Let's look at the role fats and oils play in the diet. Fats are necessary for supplying energy to the body. In addition, fats supply essential fatty acids and act as carriers for fat soluble vitamins like vitamin A, vitamin D, vitamin E, vitamin K and the carotenoids. In addition, fats have an important role to play as building blocks for various tissues and membranes, and they also play a key role in regulating numerous bodily functions.

Dietary fat is available from a variety of plant and animal sources, and most diets do contain adequate amounts of fat. Most nutrition experts recommend keeping the intake of fat to less than 20% of calories, but studies have shown that severely limiting fat intake can be dangerous. Extreme low fat diets should only be undertaking with a doctor's approval and oversight.

The type and amount of fat in the diet makes all the difference. A diet high in saturated fats, trans fats and cholesterol has been associated with a variety of ills, including heart disease, stroke and other associated diseases. In addition, many long term chronic problems, such as obesity, are associated with high levels of dietary fats.

The greatest risk of complications from excessive fat intake appears to lie with saturated fats and trans fats (fats that are solid at room temperature). One of the best ways to keep levels of saturated fat low is to limit the amount of animal fats that are consumed. These animal based fats include meats like bacon and sausage, as well as butter and ice cream. Dietary cholesterol can be limited by watching the consumption of eggs, organ meats and other foods high in cholesterol.

Food labels do make the complicated process of choosing the right fats somewhat easier. For instance, trans fats will be listed on the ingredient list of foods that contain them. In general, trans fats are found mainly in processed foods.

Some fats, such as polyunsaturated fats and monounsaturated fats, are better choices for healthy eating. Examples of these fats include canola oil and olive oil. Cooking with these lighter oils can be a big step toward a healthier diet. Polyunsaturated and monounsaturated fats are liquid at room temperature, and they have been found to have heart protecting qualities.

Many types of fish have also been found to be sources of good fat. Fish are excellent sources of omega-3 fatty acids. These omega-3's have been found to promote good health, and they may even lower cholesterol levels.

Carbohydrates are an important part of a healthy diet as well, and carbs are necessary for providing energy and many essential nutrients. Carbohydrates are found in fruits and vegetables, in grains and in milk and dairy products. It is important to choose carbohydrates carefully, however, since not all are equally healthy.

When choosing breads and cereal, for instance, try to select those made with whole grains, while avoiding the more highly refined varieties. It is also important to limit the intake of sugars, such as soda, candy and highly processed baked goods. Consuming large amounts of such high calorie, low nutrient foods, can make it very difficult to stay on a healthy diet without gaining weight.

Most Americans tend to have too much of certain elements in their diet. Sugar is one such element and salt is the other. While a basic level of sodium in the form of salt is important to proper nutrition, most people consume too much salt in their daily diet. Excess salt consumption can lead to water retention, high blood pressure and other complications. Choosing low sodium foods, and limiting the use of the salt shaker, can go a long way toward cutting levels of excess salt in the diet.

4- The importance of antioxidants in the diet

Everyone has heard the news about antioxidants and their importance to good health and proper nutrition. It seems the more scientists learn about antioxidants, the more their value and potential increases. Antioxidants have shown promise in everything from preventing heart disease to slowing the degeneration of the eyes and brain.

Antioxidants work in a fairly straightforward way. What makes them so effective is their ability to neutralize a group of highly reactive, highly destructive compounds known as free radicals.

The production of free radicals is a normal bodily process, and it is part of the process of breathing and living. Free radicals are normally neutralized by the body's natural defense system, rendering them harmless. However, anything that weakens the body's natural defenses weakens its ability to fight off these free radicals. Those weakening agents include environmental pollution, excess UV radiation and even excessive consumption of alcohol.

When free radicals are not properly neutralized, the body is left open to damage. Free radicals can damage the structure and function of cells in the body, and recent evidence suggest that free radicals contribute to the aging process and may play a role in a great many illnesses, including cancer and heart disease.

While vitamin supplements containing antioxidants such as vitamin C can be important, there is no substitute for a healthy diet. It is estimated that foods contain more than 4,000 compounds that have antioxidant qualities. Eating a healthy diet is the only way to take advantage of these antioxidant properties. In addition to the well known antioxidants like vitamin C and vitamin E, healthy foods like fruits, vegetables and whole grains also contain lots of lesser antioxidants. Scientists are only now discovering the important role these lesser known antioxidants have in keeping the body healthy.

Let's examine some of the dietary sources for the major antioxidant vitamins.

Vitamin C

Vitamin C is probably the most studied of all the antioxidant vitamins. Also known as ascorbic acid, vitamin C is a water soluble vitamin found in all bodily fluids, and it is thought to be one of body's first lines of defense against infection and disease. Since vitamin C is a water soluble vitamin, it is not stored and must be consumed in adequate quantities every day.

Good dietary sources of vitamin C include citrus fruits such as oranges and grapefruits, green peppers, broccoli and other green leafy vegetables, strawberries, cabbage and potatoes.

Vitamin E

Vitamin E is a fat soluble vitamin that is stored in the liver and other tissues. Vitamin E has been studied for its effects on everything from delaying the aging process to healing a sunburn. While vitamin E is not a miracle worker, it is an important antioxidant, and it is important that the diet contain sufficient amounts of vitamin E. Good dietary sources of this important nutrient include wheat germ, nuts, seeds, whole grains, vegetable oil, fish liver oil and green leafy veggies.

Beta-carotene

Beta-carotene is the nutrient that gives flamingos their distinctive pink color (they get it from the shrimp they eat). In the human world, beta-carotene is the most widely studied of over 600 carotenoids that have thus far been discovered. The role of beta-carotene in nature is to protect the skins of dark green, yellow and orange fruits from the damaging effects of solar radiation. Scientists believe that beta-carotene plays a similar protective role in the human body. Sources of beta-carotene in the diet include such foods as carrots, squash, sweet potatoes, broccoli, tomatoes, collard greens, kale, cantaloupe, peaches and apricots.

Selenium

Selenium is one of the most important minerals in a healthy diet, and it has been studied for its ability to prevent cell damage. Scientists see this ability to protect cells from damage as possibly important in the prevention of cancer, and selenium is being studied for possible cancer preventative properties. It is important to get the selenium you need from your diet, since large doses of selenium supplements can be toxic. Fortunately, selenium is easily found in a healthy diet. Good sources of dietary selenium include fish and shellfish, red meat, whole grains, poultry and eggs, and garlic. Vegetables grown in selenium rich soils are also good sources of dietary selenium.

5- Healthy eating with fruits and vegetables

Dietary experts recommend that every person should eat at least five servings of fruits and vegetables every day. The importance of fruits and vegetables to a healthy diet has been known for quite some time, but studies have shown that very few people eat the amount of fruits and vegetables recommended for a healthy diet.

That's a shame, since eating a sufficient number of fruits and vegetables just may be the single most effective thing you can do to improve your overall health. The five a day approach to healthy eating may be the single most important strategy you can adopt for a healthier lifestyle.

The many health benefits of eating fruits and vegetables have been established for quite some time now. Study after study has shown that a diet rich in fruits and vegetables lowers the risk of certain cancers, heart disease and other chronic diseases and conditions. Some studies have suggested that as many as 35% of cancer deaths can be attributed to diet, and that diets high in fats and low in fruits and vegetables contributes to unnecessary cancer deaths.

Fruits and vegetables have a lot of advantages besides just their nutritional importance. For one thing, they taste great and add a great deal of variety to everyday meals. Fruits and vegetables come in such a wide variety of colors, textures and flavors that they can be used in virtually every meal. Those seeking to maximize their consumption of fruits and vegetables should get into the habit of using fruits in salads, as toppings and as garnishes.

In addition to their great taste, fruits and vegetables are packed full of many essential vitamins and minerals, including many micronutrients that are not included in packaged vitamin supplements. For instance, foods like butternut squash, pumpkins, carrots, mangoes, peaches, pawpaws and green leafy vegetables are rich in beta carotene. Beta carotene is vital for healthy skin and eyes.

In addition, most varieties of fruits and vegetables contain vitamin C, another important vitamin and a strong antioxidant. Good sources of vitamin C include Brussels sprouts, citrus fruits, strawberries, broccoli, nectarines and kiwi fruit. Many fruits and vegetables, including spinach, broccoli and avocadoes, are also good sources of vitamin E, another excellent antioxidant.

Men and women alike should always strive to eat a healthy diet, but women have an extra incentive to get all the nutrition they need. Proper nutrition is essential to a healthy pregnancy, and some of the baby's biggest nutritional needs happen before the pregnancy is discovered. Folic acid is perhaps the best known essential nutrient for pregnant women. Folic acid has been proven effective at preventing a variety of birth defects, including Spina Bifida. Good dietary sources of folic acid include Brussels sprouts, broccoli, spinach and oranges. In addition, due to its importance to women of child bearing years, many common foods such as cereals and breads, are supplemented with folic acid.

In addition to their importance as source of vitamins and minerals, fruits and vegetables also provide essential dietary fiber. Adequate fiber in the diet is important in preventing heart disease and some kinds of cancer.

Another great feature of fruits and vegetables, especially to those watching their weight, is the high nutrition, low fat, low calorie nature of these foods. Fruits and vegetables contain very low levels of fats, and a diet low in fat can be quite effective for long term weight loss. In addition, fruits and vegetables contain no cholesterol, and they are lower in calories than many other types of foods.

With all these things going for them, it is no wonder so many dietary experts recommend eating a diet rich in fruits and vegetables. Not only are fruits and vegetables delicious and nutritious, but they can be quite inexpensive as well. Buying fruits and vegetables that are locally grown, and that are in season, is usually the most cost effective way to get the freshest fruits and veggies at the lowest possible cost.

This buying strategy also helps to ensure a steady stream of new fruits and vegetables every month, as some go out of season while others are just coming in. Trying a variety of different fruits and vegetables, including some you may not be familiar with, is also a great way to create exciting new dishes and prevent yourself from becoming bored with the same old

Haytham Al Fiqi

diet. Whether your goal is to lose weight or just increase your level of fitness, it is hard to go wrong with a diet rich in fruits and vegetables.

6- Tips for healthy eating with fruits and vegetables

Everyone knows the importance of a diet rich in healthy fruits and vegetables. Most people do not eat enough of these important foodstuffs, and increasing your consumption of fruits and vegetables is probably the single most effective thing you can do to improve your overall health. Eating enough fruits and vegetables does not need to be chore. After all, fruits and vegetables are delicious, easy to buy and easy to use.

In addition, fruits and vegetables are rich sources of antioxidants, which are though to play an important role in maintaining good health. Antioxidants have been studied for their effectiveness at preventing cancer, heart disease and even reversing the signs of aging. In addition, fruits and vegetables are excellent source of trace elements and other micronutrients. These important elements are not available in any vitamin pill; they must be obtained from the daily diet.

Tips for choosing the best fruits and vegetables

- ✓ When possible, choose fresh fruits possible. Fresh fruits and vegetables may contain more nutrients than frozen or dried varieties.

- ✓ Even though fresh is best, frozen and canned vegetables are great for out of season varieties. When buying canned fruits, avoid those packed in syrup and opt for those packed in water or juice.

- ✓ Choose fruits and vegetables in a variety of colors. Not only are bright, colorful fruits more attractive, but the different colors indicate different types and amounts of nutrients. For instance, yellow and orange fruits and vegetables are good sources of beta carotene, while dark green leafy vegetables are rich in vitamin C and calcium.

- ✓ Be careful when cooking vegetables. A quick steam in the microwave with minimal water added is the best way to prevent loss of nutrients when cooking.

- ✓ Keep your vegetables healthy by adding minimal butter, margarine and oil. Most vegetables can be flavored using a stock, a low fat yogurt or fresh fruit pieces.

Understanding portion sizes

We have all heard the government recommendations that we eat 5 to 10 servings of fruits and vegetables per day. This talk of servings and portions can sometimes be confusing, so let's take a look at just what a serving consists of.

A serving of a fruit or vegetable can be:

- ✓ A medium sized piece of fruit, such as an apple, banana or orange
- ✓ One large slice of a fruit like a cantaloupe, melon or pineapple
- ✓ Two pieces of small fruit, such as a kiwi fruit or plum
- ✓ One cup of strawberries, raspberries or grapes
- ✓ One half cup of fresh fruit salad
- ✓ One half cup of stewed or canned fruit
- ✓ One quarter cup of dried fruit
- ✓ One half cup of 100% pure fruit juice
- ✓ One half cup of cooked, canned or frozen vegetables
- ✓ One side salad

Unlike with many other types of foods, more is better when it comes to fruits and vegetables. When planning and preparing meals, it is important to plan ahead and include as many servings of fruits and vegetables as possible. Proper meal planning and shopping are the best ways to meet the five a day minimum recommendation for fruit and vegetable consumption.

Some tips for healthier living

- ✓ Stock the fridge with healthy snacks like celery sticks and carrots
- ✓ Keep a bowl of fruit, stocked with healthy attractive fruits like oranges, apples and bananas, on the kitchen counter and dining room table
- ✓ Drink a glass of 100% pure apple, orange or grapefruit juice every morning
- ✓ Warm up a cold day with a steaming bowl of vegetable soup
- ✓ Eat at least one salad every day. Experiment with different salad additions, like broccoli, sprouts, carrots and green peppers.
- ✓ Snack on fruits like apples and oranges. Dried fruits like apricots and raisins also make handy and nutritious snacks
- ✓ Add sprouts, cucumbers, lettuce and tomatoes to sandwiches for extra variety

- ✓ Garnish meals with chopped or grated carrots
- ✓ Strive for at least two servings of vegetables at each evening meal
- ✓ Use your creativity to create exciting vegetable stir fries for family and friends
- ✓ Spice up the grill with vegetable and fruit kebobs
- ✓ Use baked apples and pears as great low calorie desserts
- ✓ Add vegetables like carrots, cabbage, onions, lentils and peas to soups, stews and casseroles.

7- Eat a variety of foods for a healthy lifestyle

Everyone knows that variety is important when it comes to diet. Not only is eating the same foods every day boring, but it is extremely unhealthy as well. That is because each type of food contains different nutrients, and different levels of those nutrients. The best way to eat healthy is to eat a wide variety of foods from all the food groups.

It is important to eat a good combination of meats, beans, dairy products, fruits, vegetables and whole grains. All these foods contain important nutrients, and no vitamin pill in existence can provide the vast variety of nutrients your body needs every day.

Of course simply eating foods from a variety of sources is not enough. It is also important to make smart choices within those food groups. After all, nonfat yogurt and an hot fudge sundae are both dairy products! The best choice in that situation should be obvious, but other choices are more subtle.

Fortunately, the nutritional labels which are required on all packaged foods are a big help for those pursuing a healthier diet. Not only do these labels contain information on the number of calories, fat grams, etc., but they provide detailed information on the levels of many important vitamins and minerals as well.

When choosing healthy foods, small changes can have a huge impact. Simply exchanging fresh, low fat fish for higher fat meats can greatly lower the amount of fat in your diet and increase your level of health.

Replacing highly processed grains for more nutritious whole grain products can also have a great impact on healthy eating. In nutritional terms, less is often more – that is less processing and less refining. Processing and refining methods can strip many vital nutrients from foods, so choosing less refined whole grain foods is important.

Cooking techniques are also very important when maximizing the health benefits of the foods you choose. After taking the time to choose the healthiest, freshest broccoli in the supermarket, it would be quite a waste to slather that cooked broccoli with cheese and butter, for instance.

It would also be a mistake to overcook that broccoli, especially by boiling it in water for a long time. That is because vegetables can lose significant amounts of nutrients through overcooking. When preparing fresh vegetables, it is best to quickly steam them in the microwave or on the stove, using as little water as possible. Use only enough water to keep the vegetables from scorching.

When cooking potatoes, it is a good idea to eat the entire potato, including the skin. Potato skins contain significant levels of nutrients, including fiber, vitamins and minerals. Cooking a baked potato in the microwave, or on the grill, is a great way to make the skin moist and delicious. In addition, these methods of cooking minimize the need for high fat butter or sour cream to flavor the potato. In place of these high fat options, why not use a dollop of plain nonfat yogurt, or some low fat cottage cheese?

Choosing a variety of foods is important to a healthy lifestyle, but it just as important to limit the amount of certain foods. Foods high in sugar, and those high in sodium should be avoided as much as possible. That doesn't mean you can't enjoy that piece of cake or serving of potato chips as an occasional snack; it simply means limiting regular consumption of these high fat, low nutrition products.

When adopting healthier eating habits, it is important to make changes that you can stick with for the long run. After all, a healthy eating lifestyle is just that, a lifestyle. Changing your shopping, cooking and eating habits are not easy, but the many benefits make healthy eating an important habit to get into.

8- Healthy eating on a budget

For many people, a limited food budget can be a real roadblock to healthy eating. It is an unfortunate fact of life that some of the lowest priced foods, from fast food value menus to cheap potato chips, are also some of the least healthy. It is possible, however, to create excellent tasting, nutritious meals, even on a tight budget.

The key to planning and creating healthy meals on a limited budget is good forward planning and solid nutritional knowledge.

Step 1 – The shopping list

Anyone who has visited a supermarket lately knows how dangerous it is to enter the store without a shopping list in hand. Shopping without a sense of what you need – and don't need – opens you up to all manner of temptation, and most of those tempting foods are not nutritious.

In addition, picking up all those extra items can easily blow your food budget and leave you without the funds to plan those healthy, nutritious meals. A good trick is to keep a note pad near the table or refrigerator. Having the notepad within easy reach makes it easy to keep track of the foods you need to stock up on.

Step 2 – Watch those flyers

Most major food store chains publish weekly sales ads, usually as inserts in the local newspaper. Keeping track of these sales, and taking advantage of the low prices to stock up, is a great way to gather a cupboard full of healthy food. Once the pantry is full of fruits, vegetables and other healthy fare, it will be much easier to create healthy recipes the entire family will love. In addition, locally grown, in season fruits and vegetables are usually more of a bargain than out of season or shipped fruits and vegetables.

Step 3 – Stock up on staples

Essential staple foods, such as flour, rice, and pasta are frequently put on sale as loss leaders at major groceries. Stocking up on these essentials when prices are low is a great way to stretch any food budget.

Step 4 – Never shop when you are hungry

The old advice to never shop when you are hungry is definitely true. Shopping when you are hungry is a sure way to give into temptation, bust the food budget, and stock up on all the wrong foods.

Step 5 – Become a label guru

Nutritional labels contain a wealth of information, but it is up to each shopper to read those labels and understand what they mean. Nutritional labels contain complete information on not just calories and fats, but the amounts of various essential vitamins and minerals as well. It is important to know how to read labels in order to get the best nutritional bang for your food bucks.

Step 6 – Pay close attention to package sizes

Just because two cans look alike it does not mean they are. Packaging can be deceptive, so get in the habit of comparing weights when shopping for canned fruits, vegetables and other items. Also take advantage of the lower prices available on store brand and generic products.

Step 7 – Use coupons, but do it wisely

Manufacturers coupons can be a great deal when used on products you already buy. Buying something simply because you have a coupon, however, is typically not a good idea.

Step 8 – Replace meat with beans and other less costly substitutes

Eating less meat and more beans and lentils is a good way to save money on your food budget while still getting the protein you and your family need. Try experimenting with some vegetarian recipes for interesting ways to use these non meat alternatives.

In addition to the tips listed above, there are several ways that smart shoppers keep their food budgets at a minimum while preparing delicious, nutritious meals for their family every day.

One trick is to keep the refrigerator and the pantry well stocked with staple foods. Keeping a good supply of staples on hand will avoid unnecessary trips to the store and also avoid the need to buy such products when they are not on sale. When staples such as bread, flour, peanut butter, canned vegetables, etc. are on sale, be sure to stock up.

9- Healthy eating and dining out

One of the biggest challenges facing those trying to follow a healthy diet is the local restaurant. Eating out presents special challenges, such as not knowing how the food was prepared, how much fat it contains, and whether or not the healthiest ingredients were used.

Many restaurant chains, and even some fast food restaurants, have recognized the demand for healthier menu choices, and they are working hard to satisfy that demand. All too often, however, the healthy choices on a restaurant menu are limited and unappealing. It is important, therefore to pay close attention to the menu and make the healthiest choices possible.

One of the most important thing diners can do to eat healthy at restaurants is to be proactive. Diners should not be afraid to ask how a dish is prepared, or what ingredients are used in its preparation. If the server does not know, ask him or her to check with the chef. A good chef will be happy to answer such questions, and to make modifications in the recipe if needed. In addition, most restaurants will happily accommodate special needs, such as low fat or low sodium dishes. After all, the restaurant is there to serve its patrons.

Some of our favorite tips for healthy eating in restaurants include:

- One good rule of thumb to use when dining out is to order entrees that are grilled, baked or broiled. Deep fried dishes are best avoided. If you are unsure how a dish is prepared, don't be afraid to ask.

- Portion size is just as important at the restaurant as they are at home. That means ordering the petit fillet instead of the full size steak, requesting half size portions of French fries, and maybe even forgoing that tempting dessert. Choosing leaner cuts of meat or fish is also a good way to eat healthier.

- When choosing side dishes, ask if steamed vegetables are available. Steamed veggies are an excellent, low fat, low calorie choice for many diners. Vegetables that are fried, au gratin, or prepared in cream or butter sauces are best avoided.

- When ordering salad, ask if fat free choices are available. Most restaurants have several fat free or low fat varieties of salad dressing available. If no low fat option exists, request the dressing on the side so that you can control the amount that is used.

- When ordering soup, choose broth based soups, and avoid bisques or rich soups like cream of crab or cream of broccoli. A simple vegetable soup is a delicious and low fat alternative.

- Replace high fat, high calorie French fries with healthier alternatives such as fresh fruit or an unbuttered baked potato. Most restaurants will be happy to accommodate such special requests.

- In Italian restaurants, stick with the tomato based sauces and avoid cream or heavy Alfredo sauces. A simple pesto sauce without meat is a good choice for most pasta dishes.

- When dining at oriental restaurants, go with the steamed rice and stir fried vegetable entrees. Avoid the heavy sauces and request that your meal be prepared with less oil. In addition, try to choose dishes that feature less meat and more fresh vegetables.

➤ Choose a light dessert of fresh fruit or sorbet. When ordering traditional desserts, order one and share it with your dining partner.

Finally, when dining at a fast food restaurant, it is important to avoid the temptation of super sizing the meal. Fast food restaurants often make their larger portions more attractive by pricing them competitively, but a big part of healthier eating is to control portion sizes. In addition, most fast food chains now offer healthier alternatives, such as salads and baked potatoes, as well as prominently displayed nutritional information.

While dining out certainly presents challenges to those trying to enjoy a healthy lifestyle, there is no reason to forgo the pleasure of an occasional meal out. By following the guidelines listed above, and by adding some creative tips of your own, you can make dining out a healthy experience as well as a pleasant one.

10 - Healthy eating for vegetarians and vegans

Study after study has revealed the importance of a balanced diet to good health. Eating a balanced diet, one that is rich in all the various minerals and vitamins needed for a healthy body, can present quite a challenge for vegetarians and vegans.

That is because maintaining a good balanced diet in the absence of one entire food group, such as meat and poultry, can be difficult. Meat and other animal products contain significant amounts of important nutrients, such as protein, calcium and B vitamins.

Vegan diets present an even larger problem, since vegans go a step farther and eliminate dairy products and eggs as well as meat. Vegans in particular often have trouble getting the vitamin B12 they need and often must rely on vitamin supplements for this important nutrient.

Of course that does not mean that vegetarians and vegans cannot enjoy good health. Many vegetarians and vegans can and do enjoy levels of health much better than their carnivorous peers. It simply means that vegetarians need to pay somewhat closer attention to their dietary needs, and to be on the lookout for signs of dietary deficiencies. The key to a healthy vegetarian or vegan diet, as with all types of diets, is practicing moderation, eating a variety of foods, and keeping nutritional needs in balance.

One of the most frequently cited concerns by family members and friends of vegetarians and vegans is how they will get the protein they need from a diet devoid of animal flesh. However, getting sufficient protein is usually not a concern for vegetarians, since most American diets tend to contain more protein than they need.

Vegetarians who eat dairy products can get all the protein they need from dairy products, from soy based products and from beans, nuts, lentils and seeds. There are many non animal sources of protein, so most vegetarians should not have a problem getting sufficient protein.

Even vegans, who eschew all animal based products, even milk and dairy products, typically do not have a problem with protein deficiency. That is because nuts, seeds, lentils, pinto beans, split peas, soybeans, garbanzo beans, black beans, white beans, kidney beans, navy beans and many more all have lots of protein.

Vegan meals are often rich in tofu and other soy based products, and these products contain sufficient protein to meet the needs of most vegans. In addition, the many bean based vegan recipes are excellent sources of protein. For instance, a cup of cooked beans contains the same amount of protein as a two ounce serving of meat.

As with protein, nutritional deficiencies are generally of no more concern to vegetarians than they are to the general population. Vegetarians who follow a balanced, nutritious diet should have no problem meeting their daily nutritional needs.

Vegans on the other hand, are more susceptible than vegetarians to nutritional deficiencies, particularly vitamin B12, calcium and vitamin D. That is because the most common sources of these important nutrients are all animal based, either meat or dairy products.

Of these three nutrients, the hardest to replace on a vegan diet is vitamin B12. The primary sources of vitamin B12 in the diet are all animal based. For this reason, vegans are generally advised to take vitamin B12 supplement, or to eat foods that have been fortified with vitamin B12. There are a number of such foods on the market, including nutritional yeast and soy milk.

Calcium is also a concern for vegans, since the primary sources of dietary calcium are milk and other dairy products. Again, calcium fortified foods such as some soy milk and certain cereals are important to maintaining a healthy vegan diet. The same is true of vitamin D, another primarily animal based nutrient.

The bottom line is that it is possible to maintain excellent health while avoiding meat and dairy products. The key is to follow a well balanced diet, get plenty of exercise, and make smart food choices.

11- Shop smart for a healthy lifestyle

A big part of enjoying healthier eating is buying healthier foods, and that means making smart choices where it matters most – at the supermarket. Choosing the freshest, healthiest foods is an important first step toward making healthy and delicious meals your whole family will love.

In general, most supermarkets are laid out with the healthiest, most nutritious foods around the perimeter of the store. That is where most stores locate their produce section, their dairy section, their meat counter, and the like. Of course, the middle aisles of the grocery store also contain nutritious foods, such as canned and frozen vegetables, whole grain cereals and more.

And of course each shelf of the grocery store also contains both good and bad choices for healthy eating. For instance, the cereal aisle is home to both the healthy, home grain cereal, and those cereals that contain more sugar than corn. In many cases, the difference will be obvious from the packaging, while at other times you will need to read the nutritional information carefully to ensure the food is healthy for your family.

As a matter of fact, learning to read nutritional labels is one of the most important skills any health oriented shopper must learn. This government mandated labels contain a wealth of information if you know what to look for. Not only do nutritional labels contain vital information on calorie counts, fat grams and sodium content, but they contain detailed information on the percentage of each vitamin an mineral a serving contains.

When looking at nutritional labels, however, pay careful attention to the portion size listed. This is particularly important when looking at calories, fat grams and the amount of sodium. For instance, a serving of juice is generally 8 ounces, while the average juice glass at your home may be 12 or even 16 ounces. It is important to carefully look at serving size, and to do the mental calculation necessary to reflect how much of each product will actually be consumed at one sitting.

When shopping for healthy foods, it is usually better to opt for les processed foods. For instance, 100% fruit juice would be better than a fruit juice blend that may contain as little as 5% or 10% fruit juice. And plain frozen vegetables would be healthier than vegetables in a butter sauce. When shopping for meat, try to buy fresh meat whenever possible. Frozen meat products, or those already seasoned, heat and eat products, often contain unhealthy ingredients as well as preservatives.

When it comes to dairy products, it is best to buy low fat and non fat varieties when at all possible. The one exception to this rule is feeding babies and young children. Their growing bodies need the fat and calories contained in whole milk products, but adults and older children are better served by low fat alternatives.

When choosing canned soups, there are a number of fat free and low sodium varieties. Try to choose these soups for a healthier lifestyle. Other high protein, low calorie soup choices include black bean soup, lentil soup and split pea soup. These healthy soups are good sources of protein, fiber and folate.

Ethnic foods, such as Mexican and Chinese, can be excellent sources of healthy meals, and the traditional ways of preparing such foods are generally very healthy. It is important to stay as authentic as possible when choosing and preparing Mexican, Asian, Middle Eastern and Italian food. This will help guarantee both great taste and healthy eating. For instance, traditional salsa is an excellent, low calorie, and nutritious dip, and the traditional Mexican black bean dip is usually fat free.

Seasonings can be an excellent way to spice up healthy cooking without adding additional fat and calories. Herbs and spices are a great way to add zest to any meal, and starting an herb garden of your own is a great way to save both time and money while providing fresh tasting, healthy meals for your family. When buying spices in the grocery store, be especially careful about sodium content. Read the label carefully, since the first ingredient on many bottled spices is actually salt (another great reason to start that herb garden).

12- Choosing the best meat for healthy eating

Choosing the right meat and poultry products can be one of the most difficult parts of cooking and eating for better health. Meat, seafood and poultry are important sources of protein, iron, vitamins and minerals, but they are often laden with undesirable qualities such as saturated fat and cholesterol as well. Choosing the best, leanest cuts of meat is important to any health conscious shopper.

One of the most important things to know when choosing meat, seafood and poultry products is that less is often more. That means buying meat, seafood and poultry products that have been processed as little as possible. The past few years have seen quite a jump in the number of convenience foods, but these foods are often much less healthy than their fresh meat counterparts.

One reason why this is so is the need preservatives, sodium and other additives. Foods that are frozen, microwavable or ready to eat often contain large amounts of sodium, often more than you need in several days. While it is fine to keep a couple of these convenient foods on hand for quick meals, they cannot form the basis of a healthy eating lifestyle.

Fresh meat, seafood and poultry, on the other hand, does not suffer from the need to add sodium or preservatives. Buying fresh meats and seafood, and preparing it yourself, is the best way to have confidence in the nutritional quality of the food you feed your family.

Of course no discussion of fresh meat is complete without a note or two about safe handling techniques. Food borne illnesses can easily be spread through contaminated meat, poultry and seafood, and it is impossible to tell from looking if the product is contaminated. Since cooking to the proper temperature destroys these food borne pathogens, the most important thing is to keep raw meat and poultry away from foods that will not be cooked.

That means keeping things like salad bowls and bread plates well away from the area of the countertop where the meat is prepared. Any surface touched by raw meat, seafood or poultry should be thoroughly cleaned with an antibacterial solution, and separate cutting boards should be used for vegetables and meats. Following these basic food hygiene practices is the best way to protect yourself and your family from food borne illnesses.

Cutting the fat is also an important consideration when it comes to choosing meat, seafood and poultry. While most types of fish are healthy and low fat, some fish, such as salmon, can have significant fat content.

Again, the nutritional labels should be your guide.

When it comes to chicken, the best course of action is to buy skinless, boneless chicken breasts. This type of poultry is healthy, convenient and easy to use. And best of all, skinless, boneless chicken breasts are often on sale, so stock up on them when your local grocery store runs its next promotion. A good alternative for those with the time is to buy regular chicken breasts and remove the skin and bone yourself. This is often a less expensive alternative than buying the boneless, skinless chicken breast.

Ground turkey can be an excellent and lower fat alternative to ground beef, but again it is important to read the label carefully. That is because ground turkey, particularly the less expensive brands, often contain skin and fat along with the lean meat. Ground turkey breast, or a brand with a lower fat content, can be a healthier alternative. Ground turkey breast can be used in any recipe that calls for ground beef, including burritos, barbecue, tacos, chili and even hamburgers on the grill.

And of course, eating healthy does not mean giving up delicious foods like beef and pork. Lean cuts of beef and pork can be an important part of a healthy diet. Beef and pork are both excellent sources of iron, zinc and B complex vitamins, and properly prepared, lean beef and pork are nutritious as well as delicious.

And finally, there are a number of lower fat, healthier alternatives to beef and pork. Meats like buffalo, venison and emu are much lower in fat than beef, while providing the same or even higher levels of protein. The downside of these exotic meats, of course, is the price, but if you can find a local supply at a good price they are definitely worth a look.

13- Avoiding fat for healthier eating

While some fat in the diet is necessary, and it would be a mistake to try to eliminate all fat from the diet, most people simply eat too much fat. Cutting back on fat is an important part of creating a healthier diet and lifestyle.

There are a number of good reasons for cutting back on levels of dietary fat. Those reasons include:

➢ Lowering levels of dietary fat helps in weight loss and weight management. Fat contains twice as many calories per gram as protein and carbohydrates, so eating less fat usually means consuming fewer calories.

➢ Lowering fat has been shown to decrease the risk of heart disease. Dietary fat, particularly saturated fat, has been implicated as a factor in heart disease and elevated cholesterol levels.

➢ A low fat diet may help to reduce the risk of some forms of cancer. Although this matter has not been totally settled, there have been a number of studies which indicate that a diet low in fat can keep certain cancers at bay.

➢ And of course eating fewer high fat foods means that you will be able to enjoy many more low fat alternatives, such as vegetables, fruits and whole grains. Since these types of foods tend to be nutrient rich and low calorie, they can be enjoyed guilt free.

Of course cutting back on dietary fat is easier said than done, so we have compiled the list of tips for low fat healthy eating to help you get started.

✓ In place of spreads like peanut butter and full fat cream cheese, use lower fat alternatives such as low fat cream cheese, jellies, jams, fruit spreads, apple butter, mustard, low fat margarine, or low fat mayonnaise.
✓ Use high fat foods as an occasional treat, not as a dietary staple.
✓ Use reduced fat or nonfat salad dressings whenever possible. When eating out, request the salad dressing on the side so you can compare the amount used.
✓ .Instead of butter or sour cream, top baked potatoes with plain nonfat or low fat yogurt. Other delicious baked potato toppings include steamed broccoli, cottage cheese, salsa, low fat cheese and low fat or nonfat sour cream.
✓ Get creative with seasonings to add flavor without adding fat or calories. Garnishes like lemon juice, herbs, salsa or green onions are great toppings for vegetables and salads.
✓ Use high fat toppings sparingly. For instance, instead of using a tablespoon of blue cheese salad dressing, try using only a teaspoon.

✓ Avoid full fat dairy products whenever possible. Using skim milk or 2% milk instead of whole milk can make a huge difference in your daily fat intake. Likewise, low fat alternatives to ice cream, such as frozen yogurt, provide all the flavor and none of the fat.

✓ Low fat cheeses also provide a great alternative to full fat varieties. Most varieties of hard cheeses are available in low fat versions.

✓ Use low fat varieties of popular snacks. Ginger snaps, angel food cake, vanilla wafers, fig bars, jelly beans, hard candy and gum drops are all excellent choices for a sweet treat.

✓ Instead of potato chips, which are very high in fat, choose pretzels, unbuttered popcorn and other healthier alternatives.

In addition to choosing the right foods, the preparation of the foods you buy is very important to keeping fat levels as low as possible. Proper low fat food preparation starts with buying the leanest cuts of beef, pork, fish and chicken, and removing the skin and fat from chicken breasts, legs and thighs.

Broiling, backing and grilling are generally the lowest fat methods for preparing the meats and seafood you buy. Try to avoid frying foods, and if you must fry, try to use a pan that allows the excess fat and oil to drain off easily.

Healthy, low fat cooking does not have to be boring or unappetizing. There are great many excellent recipes for low fat, healthy meals that are easy to make. The most important thing is to be an educated consumer and shop carefully for the healthiest produce, meat and seafood.

14- Healthy eating for a healthy body

Healthy eating means many things to many people, and everyone has different goals for the perfect diet. The key to following a healthy diet is to find a diet you can stick with for the rest of your life. A diet should not be simply a temporary change in the way you life, eat and exercise. Rather, it should be a permanent change that you can live with day in and day out, year in and year out.

For some people, a healthy diet can be as simple as increasing the amount of fruits and vegetables in the daily diet. For others, a radical change, involving strict control of fat and cholesterol, may be required.

Of course what is needed will depend on the goal of each individual. The serious runner in search of greater conditioning will of course have different goals than the couch potato who is concerned about the possibility of heart disease.

Even though every person will different goals when it comes to healthy eating, the basic tenets of healthy eating are the same. The most important thing is to eat a good variety of foods, while eating less of the bad stuff and more of the good.

That may sound like an oversimplification, but it really is that easy. Putting that simple concept into proactive, however, is the hard part. Everyone wants to eat healthier, but there are so many temptations in today's world that healthy eating can be very difficult. The key is to make healthy choices as appealing as unhealthy ones.

One way to make healthy foods appealing is buying a wide variety of exotic fruits at the local supermarket. There are probably varieties of fruits and vegetables at your local grocery store that you never even heard of before. Why not make your next trip to the grocery store an adventure by sampling these exotic offerings?

Experimenting with new recipes is another great way to bring excitement and adventure to healthy eating. A quick perusal of your favorite low fat or healthy eating cookbook will likely present you with many fun and exciting recipes to try. Often a new cookbook, or a couple of new recipes are all it takes to spur a healthier lifestyle.

It is also important to know that eating healthier does not necessarily mean making a radical change. There are very simple things you can do, such as cutting the skin off your chicken breast, or trimming the fat from your favorite steak, that can result in significant fat reductions and health improvements. Dieters should not overlook the importance of these small changes when seeking a healthier diet.

Other examples of small changes resulting in healthier eating include:

- Replacing whole milk with skim or 2%, both in recipes and for drinking
- Snacking on sorbet or low fat frozen yogurt instead of premium ice cream
- Spraying pans with nonfat cooking spray instead of using butter or margarine
- Replacing high fat cuts of meat with leaner ones
- Eating more low fat fish and less red meat
- Using egg substitutes, the kind made from egg whites, in recipes, meals and baking

There are probably hundreds of other such tips, and they can add up to significant health improvements, whether your goal is to get fit, lose weight or improve your level of health. No matter who you are or what your current level of fitness, eating a healthier diet and losing weight may be easier than you think.

In the end, eating a healthy diet, improving your level of fitness, and managing your consumption of fat and cholesterol boils down to common sense. Depriving yourself of your favorite foods can be counterproductive to a long term dietary change. Deprivation leads inevitably to cravings, and that can start a vicious cycle of dieting and splurging.

It is best to think of healthy eating as a marathon rather than a sprint. The goal of any healthy eating program should be to make easy, lifelong changes in the way you shop, cook and dine. Only by making changes that you can follow for a lifetime will you truly be able to enjoy a healthy diet.

15- Use the five a day rule for healthy eating

The five a day rule is one of the most important rules to healthy eating. The five a day rule refers to the government's recommendation that everyone eat at least five servings a day of fruits and vegetables. At first blush, five a day seems like a reasonable goal, but most people fail to eat sufficient amounts of these important foods.

It is important to remember the many advantages of fruits and vegetables when applying the five a day rule to your own diet. For one thing, fruits and vegetables taste great, contain fewer calories than many other foods and are full of many important vitamins and minerals. In addition, fruits and vegetables are colorful and beautiful, making them great garnishes and salad toppings.

In addition, fruits and vegetables are easy to prepare, even for the busiest individual. In most cases, fresh fruits require no preparation at all, other than a quick wash and perhaps peeling.

The five a day recommendation equates to roughly two cups of fruit and two and a half cups of vegetables every day, based on the average 2,000 calorie diet. This is not a difficult goal to reach, but it is important to keep the five a day goal in mind when grocery shopping, cooking and planning meals.

One great way to get started toward a five a day lifestyle is with a delicious serving of 100% fruit juice every morning. Apple juice, grapefruit juice and orange juice are all excellent choices for both taste and nutrition.

Fruits and vegetables can also be used as garnishes for other foods. Who doesn't enjoy a sliced strawberry or banana with their morning cereal? And fruits and vegetables make great snacks as well. Whether you keep a couple of apples at your desk or a selection of carrot and celery sticks in the fridge, having fruits and vegetables readily at hand is a big part of the battle.

Of course variety is extremely important when making any change to your diet, and many dietary changes fail due to boredom. Constantly trying new varieties of fruits and vegetables is a great way to keep yourself interested in your new healthier way of eating. If you've never had kiwi fruit or asparagus, for instance, why not give it a try?

Combining attractive colors, shapes and sizes of fruits is another way to provide attractive and interesting meals for yourself and your family. Combining white grapes, red peppers and pineapple chunks can provide a delicious and attractive salad.

It is important to provide constant variety when implementing the five a day plan, particularly if you are cooking for a family. Try making some interesting new dishes, such as veggie pizza, made with fresh vegetables and whole wheat pizza crust, a fresh vegetable wrap, vegetable stir fry or pasta with fresh vegetables.

For those who think they are too busy to incorporate five servings of fruits and vegetables a day into their diet, there is help available. The many ready to eat, prepackaged salad kits on the market make it easier than ever to create a healthy salad on the go. Just keep a bottle of your favorite low fat or nonfat salad dressing on hand and you can enjoy a healthy salad anywhere and anytime.

Even fast food restaurants have made it easier than every to eat healthy, with every major chain now offering at least a few healthy menu items. In addition, most grocery chains offer fresh salad bars where you can create your own healthy lunch even if you're pressed for time.

When creating your five a day healthy lifestyle, remember that fruits and vegetables make great snacks. An apple, orange or banana provides both great taste and excellent nutrition. In addition, the natural sugars contained in fruits do not provide the sugar high/sugar crash scenario all parents are familiar with.

Topping meals and salads with additional fruits and vegetables is a great way to enhance your new five a day lifestyle. Strips of green and red peppers, broccoli florets, sliced carrots and cucumbers are all great additions to pasta and potato salads. And of course carrots, spinach, apple slices, orange slices, nectarines, pineapples and raisins are all great additions to any salad.

In addition, adding fresh fruits to foods you already eat is a great way to make such foods part of your new lifestyle. Adding berries, bananas or oranges to cereal and yogurt is a great way to make sure you meet your five a day goal every day.

16- Cooking tips for healthier eating

Most people have heard that the new government guidelines recommend that all Americans eat at least five servings of fruits and vegetables every day. While that may seem like a lot, it is actually easier than you think to consume all the fruits and vegetables you need each and every day.

Learning to cook with the many fruits and vegetables available at the local grocery store is an essential skill, and it is very important for those who hope to reach the five a day guideline set down by the USDA.

Just about everyone uses a microwave these days, and microwave ovens can make cooking with vegetables and fruits easy and fun. Using a microwave pressure cooker or microwave proof bowl is a great way to quickly steam veggies. Cooking vegetables this way allows them to retain their all important nutrients.

The microwave is also a great way to cook baked potatoes, and micro waved baked potatoes retain more of their natural moisture, therefore needing less of that fat laden butter and sour cream. Combining free steamed broccoli with that great baked potato gets you almost halfway to your goal of five servings of vegetables and fruits per day.

The grill is another great way to meet your goal of five servings of fruits and vegetables every day. Why not use green peppers, red peppers and pineapple chunks to create delicious and colorful vegetable kebobs? Whether served with lean cuts of beef or by themselves, vegetable kabobs are a great treat for the whole family. Vegetables are best grilled over medium hot coals.

Those with a blender handy can make some wonderful smoothies with the great fresh fruit from the grocery store. Delicious smoothies can be made using peaches, nectarines, crushed ice and fruit juice.

For a quick fruit salad, simply open a can of mandarin oranges, add a banana, an apple, and strawberries, blueberries or raisins. The total preparation time for this great fruit salad is all of five minutes.

Fruit skewers are even easier to make than grilled vegetable skewers. Fruit skewers can easily be made by stacking strawberries, melon slices, grapes and chunks of pineapples. A great dip can be made using nonfat plain or vanilla yogurt.

Another great way to meet your five a day fruit and vegetable goal is by making your own healthy salsa. There are some great recipes for salsa on the internet, using such great and healthy ingredients as tomatoes, avocados, red onions, mangoes, cilantro and lime.

For those looking for a fun way to enjoy fruits and vegetables, why not make some popsicles? Popsicles are not just for kids anymore, and pouring fruit or vegetable juice into a popsicle mold is a great way to make a delicious and nutritious snack. In addition, these healthy popsicles are a great way to get the kids interested in eating healthy at an early age. Since eating habits picked up in childhood can last a lifetime, that is very important.

In addition to these great fruit and vegetable serving suggestions, there are other ways to create memorable meals using your five a day criteria. For instance, adding broccoli florets, slices of carrots, cucumber slices, green peppers and red peppers is a great way to add crunch and zest to a bland pasta salad.

A plain old green salad can be perked up by including colorful fruits and vegetables like carrots, spinach leaves, tangerine slices, nectarines, grapes, slices of apples, pineapples and raisins. Not only to these additions add beauty and drama to any salad, but they get you closer to your goal of five servings of fruits and vegetables a day.

For a simple, inexpensive and nutritious salad dressing, try such novel approaches as fruit juices, flavored vinegars and home grown herbs. Creating great tasting salads is very important for healthy eating, and avoiding high fat salad dressings is an important consideration for anyone concerned about their health.

Another great way to ensure you eat plenty of vegetables and fruits is to add those vegetables and fruits to the foods you already eat. That can be as simple as adding green peppers and red peppers to your pizza, adding pineapple chunks to your shish kebobs, adding bananas to your cereal or adding blueberries to your daily serving of yogurt.

Eat Healthier: Tips for healthy eating

17- Eating well on a tight budget

Just about everyone wants to eat better, but budgetary constraints sometimes make healthy eating a difficult goal. It is important, however, to buy the healthiest food you can afford, whether you are cooking only for yourself or for a growing family.

One fun and easy way to cook healthy food while still saving money is to grow your own herbs and spices. Unlike a vegetable garden, that can take up lots of space and involve a lot of work, a simple herb garden can be easily grown in a windowsill or similar small space. There are kits available for just a few dollars that contain the seeds, pots and other items needed to start an herb garden, or you can save even more money by buying the seeds and planters yourself.

Cooking with herbs and spices is a great way to enjoy healthy cooking on a budget. Spices and herbs are a great way to flavor dishes without the need for heavy sauces, butter or other high fat preparations. Growing your own herbs give the grower a great deal of control over those herbs. This is important, since many prepared herbs and spices contain large amounts of sodium.

Another excellent way to save money while still eating a healthy diet is to buy fresh fruits and vegetables when they are in season in your local area. Buying locally grown produce is often the best way to guarantee freshness and quality, and in season produce is generally less expensive since it does not need to be shipped hundreds or even thousands of miles.

Watching the sales at the local grocery stores is important to everyone, but it is particularly important to those who are trying to eat right on a limited budget. Using grocery store sales to stock up on such important staples as whole grain cereals, breads and whole wheat flour is a great way to make even the most limited food budget stretch a bit further.

Using coupons is another great way to make a food budget stretch. Cutting coupons is a great way to save money on products you already buy, as is signing up for various frequent buyer programs and other money savings opportunities.

In addition to manufacturers coupons, many grocery store chains offer customer loyalty cards which allow their customers to save money on products they buy regularly. These grocery store loyalty programs often print coupons for products customers have bought in the past, and they can be great ways to save significant amounts of money. Since most of these programs are free, there is really no downside to their use.

Stocking up on meats, seafood and poultry during store sales is another great way to save significant amounts of money. Buying a second hand chest freezer may be a good investment, particularly for those people with large families to feed. Having a large freezer space allows customers to take advantage of grocery store sales and stock up on chicken, beef, lamb, fish and pork when they are on sale.

Careful meal planning is another great way to save money while still providing healthy meals for yourself and your family. Planning meals well ahead of time allows you to take advantage of what is already in your freezer in order to create delicious, nutritious meals without spending any additional money.

One great thing about most fruits, vegetables and beans is their low cost. Another great feature of these staples is their high nutritional value. Combining these two important features is a great way to make your budget stretch while providing your family with nutritious, healthy foods.

For instance, why not make that expensive skirt steak go further by interspersing chunks of expensive beef with chunks of inexpensive pineapples or green peppers. Not only will you get twice as much food for your money, but you will enjoy a healthier meal as well.

No matter what strategies you choose to make your food budget stretch when cooking healthy meals, we think you will find that cooking healthy is worth any sacrifice it may require. Healthy cooking will pay big dividends in increased health and fitness, as well as increased energy levels.

18- Enjoy a variety of vegetables for healthy living

Eating healthy is important for everyone, and one of the most important keys to eating a better diet is eating more fruits and vegetables. Many people are unsure how to use vegetables more effectively as part of their diet, but it may be easier than you think to provide yourself and your family with healthy, nutritious meals at a great prices.

One way to create wonderful meals that are healthier than ever is to take a stroll through the produce section of your local grocery store. Most major grocery store chains have huge produce sections, containing a wonderful variety of fruits and vegetables from all corners of the world.

Trying a variety of different fruits and vegetables is a great way to keep your meals interesting and exciting in addition to nutritious. It is all too easy to become bored when trying to follow a healthy diet, and boredom can lead people to abandon their healthy habits. Avoiding diet burnout is important to the long term survival of even the most sensible eating plan.

So if you've never had vegetables like collard greens, asparagus or kale before, why not give them a try. Not only can trying new things allow you to make great new discoveries, but it can increase your level of fitness as well. Leafy green vegetables like spinach, broccoli and kale are rich sources of many important vitamins, minerals and other micronutrients.

Another great way to increase the variety of vegetables you enjoy is to combine fresh, frozen and canned vegetables. While fresh vegetables are generally better and healthier, frozen and canned vegetables can be great alternatives for when the fresh varieties are out of season.

One of the best things about fresh fruits and vegetables is the great variety of flavors, colors and textures available. Eating a variety of different colored vegetables and fruits does much more than provide much needed variety. It also provides a great variety of nutrients. For instance, yellow and orange fruits and vegetables tend to be very high in beta carotene, while green leafy vegetables are often great sources of calcium and other important nutrients. So why not spice up your plain old green salad with a splash of color in the form of yellow peppers or orange carrot slices?

Many people wrongly think that they can make up for a crappy diet by using vitamin and mineral supplements. This mistaken belief is apparently very widespread, since sales of these supplements continue to break records.

When considering vitamin and mineral supplements, however, it is important to remember that foods contain many different minerals, trace elements and other micronutrients. That means that for every nutrient that has been discovered and synthesized, there may be ten, twenty or more of these micronutrients that have yet to be fully understood. That is why no vitamin supplement, no matter how complete, can truly replace a healthy, balanced diet.

In addition, vitamin and mineral supplements are quite a bit more expensive than a good selection of vegetables and fruits, and not nearly as tasty.

When changing your diet and eating for a healthier lifestyle, it is important to educate yourself about eating right, and go choose the right fruits and vegetables for your tastes. After all, the best diet is the one you can follow for the rest of your life.

One of the best ways to start eating a healthy diet is to choose the freshest fruits and vegetables. Not only do fresh fruits and vegetables taste better, but they are less expensive and more nutritious as well. Choosing a variety of in season fruits and vegetables every week is a great way to enjoy healthy and varied meals.

Of course your favorite fruits and vegetables will not always be in season, so it will sometimes be necessary to supplement those fresh fruits and vegetables with canned and frozen varieties. When choosing canned fruits, try to avoid those packed in syrup; choose canned fruits packed in fruit juice or water instead. They will be healthier and contain less sugar.

Adding fresh fruit, such as apple slices, mandarin oranges, nectarines and the like is a great way to make plain salads more interesting and more delicious. Combining fruits and vegetables is a great way to enhance your nutrition as well.

19- Variety – your key to a healthy diet

It has been said that variety is the spice of life, and that is certainly true when trying to eat a healthy diet. No one likes to eat the same thing day after day, and boredom is the enemy of a healthy diet.

Fortunately for those trying to follow a healthy diet, there is plenty of variety to be had in healthy foods. In addition to the hundreds of varieties of fruits and vegetables available at the average grocery store, there is a wide variety of beans, lentils, nuts, meat, dairy products, fish and poultry. There is no need for boredom to set in when pursuing a healthier lifestyle.'

The key to enjoying a variety of foods while eating healthy is to plan meals carefully and be sure to use the many varieties of foods that are available. Using a combination of fresh fruit, vegetables, meats and whole grains, it is possible to create a fresh, exciting and healthful meal every day of the week.

Nutritionists often stress the importance of a varied diet, both for nutritional and psychological reasons. A varied diet is essential for good health, since different types of foods contain different types of nutrients. And following a varied diet is important to your psychological well being as well, since feeling deprived of your favorite foods can lead you to give up your healthy lifestyle.

It is much better to continue eating the foods you like, but to eat them in moderation. Instead of giving up that juicy bacon, for instance, have it as an occasional treat, perhaps pairing it with an egg white omelet instead of a plateful of scrambled eggs. As with everything else in life, good nutrition is a tradeoff.

It is important for everyone to eat foods from the five major food groups each and every day. The five food groups identified by the USDA include grains, vegetables, fruits, milk and dairy and meat and beans. Each of these food groups contains specific nutrients, so it is important to eat a combination of these foods to ensure proper levels of nutrition.

Of course simply choosing foods from the five food groups is not enough. After all a meal from the five food groups could include cake, candied yams, avocados, ice cream and bacon. Although all five food groups are represented, no one would try to argue that this is a healthy day's menu. Choosing the best foods from within each group, and eating the less healthy foods in moderation, is the best way to ensure a healthy and varied diet.

For instance, choosing healthy, lean meats is a great way to get the protein you need without consuming unnecessary fat and calories. And removing fat and skin from chicken is a great way to eliminate extra fat and calories.

When choosing breads and cereals, it is usually best to choose those that carry the whole grain designation. Whole grains, those that have not been overly refined, contain greater nutritional qualities and fewer sugars.

In addition, many grains and cereals are fortified with additional vitamins and minerals. While this vitamin fortification is important, it should be seen as a bonus, not as a substitute for a proper diet. Many foods are supplemented with important nutrients such as calcium (essential for strong bones and teeth) and folic acid (important in preventing birth defects).

Substituting healthier foods for less healthy ones is a cornerstone of a healthy diet. For instance, substituting lean cuts of meat for fattier ones, and substituting skinless chicken or turkey breast for less healthy drumsticks, is a great way to maximize nutrition without sacrificing good taste.

No matter what your reason for following a healthy diet, or what your ultimate fitness goals may be, you will find that a good understanding of nutrition will form the basis of your healthy diet. Understanding how the various food groups work together to form a healthy diet will go a long way toward helping you meet your ultimate fitness goals. Whether your goal is to run a marathon, lose ten pounds or just feel better, knowledge is power, and nutritional knowledge will power your diet for the rest of your life.

20- Fats and carbohydrates – their place in a healthy diet

Lately it would seem that fats and carbohydrates have both gotten a bad rap. First it was fat that was the culprit in all dietary ills, and low fat diets were all the rage. Then the two switched places, with carbohydrates being the bad guys and fat reigning supreme.

As with most extremes, the truth lies somewhere in the middle. There is no such thing as a bad food, only bad dietary choices. While some foods are naturally better for you than others, there is no reason that all foods cannot be enjoyed in moderation. After all, the most successful diet is not one that you can follow for a day, a week or even a year. On the contrary, the only successful diet and nutrition program is one that you will be able to follow for a lifetime.

Both fats and carbohydrates play an important role in nutrition, and both are important to a healthy diet. It would be impossible and unwise to eliminate all fat from the diet, since fat is important for the production of energy, and for carrying valuable fat soluble vitamins like vitamin D, vitamin E and vitamin K, throughout the body. In addition, fat plays a vital role in regulating various bodily functions.

Even though some fat is essential to a healthy body, too much fat can be harmful. Excessive levels of dietary fats have been implicated in heart disease, stroke, high cholesterol levels and even some cancers. Most nutritionists recommend limiting daily fat intake to less than 20% of calories, although taking that level lower than 10% is not recommended.

Of course not all fats are created equal, and some fats are more harmful than others. Saturated fats and trans fats are generally understood to be more harmful in the diet than polyunsaturated and monounsaturated fats. These lighter fats, like canola oil and olive oil, should form the basis of cooking a healthier diet.

Keeping saturated fats and trans fats to a minimum is important to a healthy diet. Trans fats, which are solid at room temperature, are most often found in highly processed foods like cookies, cakes and other baked goods. In addition, trans fats are often found in fried foods and in salty snacks like potato chips. While these foods are fine in moderation, it is best to avoid large quantities of such snacks.

One additional word here about good fats – yes there are such things, and one of the most powerful of these are the so called omega-3 fatty acids. These fats are most often found in fish, and they have shown great promise in preventing and even reversing heart disease and high cholesterol levels.

When limiting your daily intake of fat and cholesterol, it is good to have an understanding of nutritional labels. These government mandated labels can be a huge help to those who take the time to read and understand them. Not only do nutritional labels provide valuable information on calories, fat content and sodium, but they provide valuable information about the most important vitamins and minerals as well.

Like fats, carbohydrates are found in a variety of different foods, some healthier than other. For instance, both Twinkies and whole wheat bread are sources of carbohydrates, but while one can form the basis of a healthy diet, the other is best used as an occasional snack.

In addition to cereals and breads, carbohydrates are also present in fruits and vegetables and in milk and other dairy products. Carbohydrates and fats are both important to a healthy, varied diet.

As with many products, less is often more when it comes to choosing foods rich in carbohydrates. For instance, less refined whole grain bread is generally more nutritious than white bread which has gone through a greater amount of refining. That is because the refining process tends to reduce nutrient content over time.

Of course, there are some elements in the diet that should be limited. Two of these elements are sugar and salt. Most Americans consume too much salt and sugar, and this has led to epidemics of obesity, diabetes, heart disease and other ills. Limiting sugar and salt, while choosing good fats and unrefined carbohydrates, is a great way to maximize the nutritional value of the foods you eat.

21- Get your antioxidants the natural way – through your diet

You may have about the importance of antioxidants in the diet, and their possible role in fighting a variety of illnesses, including some kinds of cancer, age related degeneration and heart disease.

You could also be forgiven for thinking that antioxidant vitamins are things that come in pills, powders and capsules. The marketing of antioxidant vitamin supplements, such as vitamin A, vitamin C and vitamin E, is intense and relentless. While vitamin supplements can be helpful, however, the majority of antioxidant vitamins should come from food, not from vitamin supplements.

It is important to understand how antioxidant vitamins work to protect the body from harm. Antioxidants work by combining with and neutralizing harmful elements known collectively as free radicals. Free radicals are produced naturally by the body, as a consequence of a number of natural bodily processes. Most of the time, the body is able to neutralize and eliminate these free radicals on its own.

However, stresses such as environmental pollution, a weakened immune system, UV radiation and alcohol consumption can lower the body's ability to fight these free radicals.

Excessive free radicals in the human body can cause damage to the structure and function of the various organs and systems in the body. Recent studies have implicated free radicals in a number of diseases, including cancer and heart disease. In addition, free radicals are thought to play a significant role in the aging process.

It is estimated that foods contain some 4,000 different compounds that have antioxidant qualities. Since only a small number of these compounds have been identified, and a lesser amount yet have been synthesized, it is easy to see why it is so hard for vitamin supplements to replace a healthy diet. Healthy, antioxidant containing foods like fruits, vegetables and whole grains, contain a variety of vitamins, minerals, trace elements and other micronutrients in addition to the antioxidants that have been identified by science.

There are many major vitamins that have been found to have strong antioxidant qualities. Perhaps the most well known, and the most studied, of these antioxidant vitamins is vitamin C. Vitamin C, also known as ascorbic acid, is water soluble and is found in all the tissues and fluids of the body. Since vitamin C is not stored in the body, it is important that everyone's diet contain plenty of vitamin C.

Good sources of vitamin C in the diet include citrus fruits like oranges and grapefruits, green peppers, broccoli, strawberries, cabbage and potatoes. Dark green leafy vegetables are also good sources of vitamin C.

Vitamin E is another popular member of the antioxidant family, and it is thought to play an important role in protecting the body from aging. Vitamin E may not be the cure all wonder that it was once thought to be, but it is still an important protector of the body.

Good sources of dietary vitamin E include nuts, seeds, wheat germ, whole grain breads, vegetable oil, fish oil and dark green leafy vegetables.

Beta carotene is also an important antioxidant vitamin, and it is important to a number of bodily processes. The role of beta carotene in the natural world is to protect the skins of yellow and orange vegetables and fruits from the damaging rays of the sun. It is believed that beta carotene plays the same sort of role in human nutrition. That is, beta carotene is thought to be important in protecting people from the damage caused by environmental pollution, UV rays, etc.

Beta carotene rich foods include yellow and orange vegetables and fruits such as carrots, yellow squash, sweet potatoes, cantaloupes, peaches and apricots. In addition, dark green leafy vegetables such as collard greens and broccoli, and fruits like tomatoes, also contain significant levels of beta carotene.

Selenium is an important mineral thought to share many traits with antioxidants. Selenium in particular has been studied for its ability to prevent and reverse cell damage. Scientists continue to focus on this cell protecting ability as a possible cancer fighter.

Selenium is one good example of why it is important to get the nutrients you need from food, not from vitamin supplements. High levels of selenium can be toxic, so supplementation is not recommended. Foods high in selenium, such as fish, shellfish, red meat, poultry, eggs, garlic and whole grains, however, are recommended. In addition to these sources of selenium, fruits and vegetables that are grown in selenium rich soils are also good sources of this important mineral.

Eat Healthier: Tips for healthy eating

22- Getting the most from fruits and vegetables in the diet

Every nutritional expert stresses the importance of fruits and vegetables in the diet. Fruits and vegetables are one of those rare cases in which more is better, and the new dietary guidelines recommend that everyone eat at least five servings of fruits and vegetables every day.

Unfortunately for the health of America, most people do not eat sufficient quantities of these important nutrients. That is too bad, since increasing the amount of fruits and vegetables you consume may well be the most important and easiest dietary change anyone can make.

The health benefits of eating large quantities of fruits and vegetables has long been established, and study after study has shown that eating fruits and vegetables is a great way to increase your level of fitness and nutrition.

Fruits and vegetables have been studied for their role in preventing a number of diseases, including heart disease, stroke, aging related conditions and even some forms of cancer. Some studies have shown that as many as 35% of all cancers are related to diet, and diets high in fat and low in fruits and vegetables seem to make many people especially vulnerable to such illnesses.

Of course the appeal of fruits and vegetables is not limited to their health benefits. After all, fruits and vegetables are delicious as well as nutritious, and the variety of shapes, sizes, colors and textures mean that there are fruits and vegetables to suit virtually every taste.

Fruits and vegetables are also a great source of antioxidant vitamins, including vitamins A, C and E. Antioxidant vitamins are thought to play a vital role in protecting the body from harm caused by environmental pollution, UV rays and other modern hazards.

In addition, many fruits and vegetables are chock full of important nutrients like beta carotene. Beta carotene is the nutrient that gives those pink flamingos their distinctive color, and it is found in many orange and yellow fruits and vegetables. Foods such as mangoes, peaches, carrots, pumpkins and butternut squash are particularly rich in beta carotene.

While fruits and vegetables are important to everyone, they are just as important to those not yet born. Women of child bearing age should be sure to consume plenty of foods rich in folic acid. That is because folic acid is important in preventing many birth defects, such as spina bifida. Since sufficient folic acid is important to the proper development of the baby, it is important that the mother's body contain plenty of folic acid, even before she knows she is pregnant. Good sources of dietary folic acid include vegetables like Brussels sprouts, broccoli and spinach and citrus fruits like oranges.

Fruits and vegetables are important sources of dietary fiber in addition to being great sources of vitamins, minerals and trace elements. Proper levels of fiber are important in the prevention of heart disease and even some types of cancer.

In addition, fruits and vegetables are usually low in calories, while at the same time they are very high in nutritional values. Low fat, high nutrition, low calorie foods are hard to find, but the world of fruits and vegetables is full of such foods. In addition, fruits and vegetables contain no cholesterol or fat.

With all these advantages, it is easy to understand why fruits and vegetables are so important to a good, balanced diet. In addition, fruits and vegetables are among the least expensive types of foods. Locally grown, in season fruits and vegetables can be a great value, and most grocery store chains run regular specials on locally grown produce.

Buying locally grown, fresh fruits and vegetables is also a great way to ensure a steady supply of new tastes, colors and textures. There are literally hundreds of varieties of fruits and vegetables, and eating a variety of produce is a great way to keep boredom from setting in and sabotaging your diet.

23- Citrus Fruits and Healthy Eating

Citrus fruits have long been known to have many health benefits. In the days of the first ocean crossings, sailors often became sick with scurvy due to vitamin C deficiencies caused by a lack of citrus fruits. Even though vitamin C deficiency is no longer such a problem, many people do not eat enough citrus fruits.

That is a shame, since citrus fruits are among the most delicious, and most nutritious, fruits available. Whether you have a grapefruit at breakfast or an orange at lunch, adding more citrus to your diet can do wonders for your healthy eating program.

Of course citrus fruits are not limited to the standard oranges and grapefruits. Most major grocery stores have an endless variety of citrus fruits on their shelves, including pineapples, tomatoes, lemons kumquats, mandarin oranges, tangerines, and lemons.

Everyone knows that citrus fruits have large amounts of vitamin C to offer, but many citrus fruits have significant levels of other important nutrients, such as potassium, as well. Let's take a closer look at what citrus fruits have to offer.

Vitamin C

Vitamin C is the first thing that comes to mind when most people think of citrus fruits, and it is true that most citrus fruits are simply loaded with this important vitamin. Vitamin C is perhaps the most studied of all vitamins, and it has shown promise in shortening the duration of colds, helping wounds heal faster, and protecting the body from the damaging effects of free radicals.

Vitamin C is essential for healthy skin and gums, and since vitamin C is a water soluble vitamin, sufficient quantities must be consumed every day. Unlike fat soluble vitamins, vitamin C is not stored in the body. That is why eating at least a few servings a day of citrus fruits and other vitamin C rich foods is so important. Luckily, getting the recommended daily amount of vitamin C is not difficult, since a single orange contains 150% of the government's recommended daily allowance of vitamin C.

Fiber

Fiber content is often overlooked as a benefit of citrus fruits. After all, most people picture cereals and grains when they think of fiber. Even so, citrus fruits are a good source of dietary fiber, including the all important soluble fiber. Fiber plays a vital role in digestion, and studies have indicated it may help to reduce levels of cholesterol in the blood and even reduce the risk of some kinds of cancer.

Folate (folic acid)

Folate, or folic acid as it is also known, plays a vital role in early pregnancy, so all women of child bearing age are encouraged to consume adequate amounts of this important nutrient. That is because one of the most critical times in a pregnancy takes place before the woman knows she is pregnant.

In addition to its importance in preventing many neural tube birth defects, folic acid also aids in the production of mature red blood cells and helps to prevent anemia. Citrus fruits are an excellent source of folic acid.

Potassium

Oranges are particularly high in potassium, as are non citrus fruits like bananas. Potassium is vital to maintaining a proper fluid balance in the body, and for transmitting signals between nerve cells. Potassium levels can be affected by excess caffeine consumption and by dehydration, so it is important to consume adequate levels of potassium every day.

With all these things going for them, it is easy to see why citrus fruits are so important to the diet. No matter what your ultimate fitness goal, a diet rich in citrus fruits will help to get you off to the right start. And with the many varieties of citrus fruits to choose from, it is easy to spice things up and bring variety to your healthy eating plan.

24- The importance of fiber to a healthy diet

When it comes to eating healthy and enjoying a healthier lifestyle, it is hard to overstate the importance of fiber in the diet. Even though fiber is most associated with grains, rice and breads, it is important to remember that fruits and vegetables also contain significant amounts of dietary fiber. In fact, the need for fiber is just one more reason to eat your fruits and vegetables every day.

In order to understand why dietary fiber is so important, it is a good idea to know what fiber is and what role it plays in digestion. Simply put, dietary fiber is the portion of food that the human body cannot digest. Fiber is found in foods of plant origin only; there is no fiber in meat and dairy products. Fiber plays an important role in the digestion of food, and in the elimination of waste products as they travel through the body.

Good sources of dietary fiber include grains, cereals, legumes, lentils, nuts, seeds, fruits and vegetables. As we said before, meats and dairy products do not contain any dietary fiber, so it is important to eat some plant based foods ever day to get the fiber you need.

Soluble vs. insoluble

Not all fiber is the same, and fiber comes in two forms – soluble and insoluble. All plant materials contain both types of fiber, but some sources contain more of one than the other. Eating a variety of foods rich in fiber every day will ensure you get adequate levels of both soluble and insoluble fiber.

Insoluble fiber is important in keeping people regular, and it has shown promise as well in the prevention of some types of colon and rectal cancers. Insoluble fiber is mainly found in wheat brain, some types of vegetables and in whole grain products. Some vegetables rich in insoluble fiber include carrots, peas and broccoli. The skins of fruits are also rich in insoluble fiber.

Soluble fiber, on the other hand, has shown promise in reducing levels of cholesterol in the blood, and at reducing the rate at which glucose enters the bloodstream. Soluble fiber is abundant in dried peas, lentils, beans, barley, oat bran, and in many fruits and vegetables.

How much fiber is enough

Many people are unsure just how much dietary fiber they need every day, but most dietitians recommend that women consume between 21 and 25 grams of dietary fiber per day. For men, the recommendation is 30 to 38 grams of fiber each day.

Of course, that is easier said that done, and it is important to know which foods are high in fiber in order to boost your daily fiber consumption. In the case of packaged foods like breads and crackers, the fiber content will be listed as part of the nutritional label. In the case of fruits and vegetables, there are charts which show the fiber content of an average size piece. Some grocery stores post this information, and it is also widely available on the internet.

When increasing dietary fiber, it is best to make the increase gradual. A sudden jump in dietary fiber can lead to bloating, gas and abdominal discomfort. In addition, it is important to drink plenty of fluids, especially water, in order for fiber to have the best effect. When choosing breads and cereals, it is best to go with healthier whole grains. In general, the less processing, the healthier the foods.

Eating the skins of fruits and vegetables is a great way to increase dietary fiber. Many people like to make fruit shakes and smoothies that use the skins of their favorite fruits. This makes a delicious and nutritious way to increase fiber consumption. In addition, keeping a variety of fiber rich foods, such as apples, nuts, seeds and bran muffins, around for snacks is a great idea.

And finally, eating a wide variety of foods will ensure that you get plenty of fiber, as well as the vitamins, minerals, and trace elements that make a balanced diet so important.

25- Keeping fat low for a healthier eating lifestyle

Everyone has heard about the importance of keeping the level of fat in the diet to a minimum. While some fat in the diet is necessary, most Americans eat far too many fatty foods. Fats do play a vital role in the diet, including in the absorption of important fat soluble vitamins like vitamin A, vitamin D, vitamin E and vitamin K. These vitamins are stored in fatty tissues, and dietary fat aids in this process.

Too much fat in the diet, however has been linked to high cholesterol, heart disease and even some kinds of cancers. Eating less fat, especially less saturated fat and trans fats, is an important part of adopting healthier eating habits.

For this reason, it is important to use foods that are high in dietary fats as an occasional snack or treat, and not as a staple of the diet. Many meats are high in fat, so it is important to choose lean cuts of meat whenever possible, and to trim excess fat from steaks and chops. Even some poultry can be high in fat, and for this reason, removing the skin from chicken, and avoiding fatting dark meat, is a good practice to follow.

When planning your healthy eating lifestyle, it is important to remember that fat, whether from plant or animal sources, contains more than twice the number of calories per gram as protein or carbohydrates. Experts recommend that people limit the amount of dietary fat to no more than 30% of total calories. Since fat is so calorie dense, simply cutting back on the number of fat grams per day can result in a significant lowering of daily calorie consumption. That is why low fat diets are so effective as weight loss plans.

Some fats are worse than others – there are both saturated and unsaturated varieties of fats. Unsaturated fats further break down into monounsaturated and polyunsaturated varieties. In general, unsaturated fats are healthier than saturated fats. Saturated fats have been shown to raise levels of cholesterol in the blood more than unsaturated fat. Reducing the level of saturated fats to fewer than 10 percent of daily calories is a proven way to lower levels of cholesterol in the blood.

Meat, milk, dairy products and eggs are the main sources of saturated fats in moth diets. In addition, many baked goods are also rich in saturated fats, since they are often cooked in fatty oils and contain eggs and other fatty ingredients.

When cooking with oils, it is important to choose the healthiest ones. Olive oil and canola oil both use unsaturated fats, and they tend to be very useful in healthy cooking. There are even such things as good fats. In particular, omega-3 oils found in fish are good sources of these fats. Omega-3 oils have been shown to have a protective effect on the heart, and in lowering blood cholesterol levels.

Listed below are some of our favorite tips for keeping dietary fat and cholesterol as low as possible:

- ✓ Use fatty cooking oils sparingly
- ✓ Make fatting foods an occasional treat, not an everyday source of nutrition
- ✓ Pay close attention to the nutritional labels on packaged foods and meats. These labels provide valuable information on fat content, calorie content and nutritional quality
- ✓ Eat a diet rich in low fat foods like whole grains, fruits and vegetables
- ✓ Choose low fat varieties of your favorite foods whenever possible. There are excellent nonfat varieties of milk, dairy products, baked goods, and more
- ✓ Choose lean cuts of meat whenever possible, and trim additional fat before cooking and serving

Cutting fat is not easy, but the many benefits of a low fat diet make it a very worthwhile change. There are few dietary changes that impart as many health benefits as does cutting the fat from your diet. A few changes here and there can add up to a huge change and make a real difference in your health.

26- Choosing low fat high fiber foods for a healthy diet

Raising the level of dietary fiber, while lowering the amount of fat in your diet, is one of the most effective changes you can make, both in terms of weight loss and overall health and fitness. Unfortunately, most people consume too much fat and not enough fiber, and reversing that trend can be difficult even for the most motivated.

A good place to start is by knowing which foods are highest in dietary fiber. Eating a diet rich in these foods is a good way to boost fiber while lowering fat and other negative dietary elements.

When boosting the amount of fiber in the diet, however, it is best to start gradually in order to let your body adjust. An abrupt change in the amount of fiber in the diet can lead to cramps, abdominal pain, bloating and gas.

Among the highest fiber foods are cooked legumes (including dried peas and beans), dried fruits, nuts, sesame seeds, sunflower seeds, and berries.

These foods all contain more than six grams of fiber per serving.

Foods which contain from four to six grams of fiber per serving include a baked potato (with the skin), apples, pears, barley, brown rice, bran muffins, lima beans, snow peas, green peas and sweet potatoes.

Further down the scale at two to four grams per serving are vegetables, citrus fruits, whole wheat bread, rye bread and melons. These foods are still good sources of fiber, but you will need to eat more of them to get the full effect. That's fine, though, since they are healthy, nutritious foods in many ways.

In order to enjoy healthier eating habits for life, it is important to make fundamental changes in the way you shop, cook and eat. A diet should be more than a temporary change in eating habits; a true dietary change must be one you can follow for a lifetime.

When doing the weekly grocery shopping, get into the habit of hitting the produce section first. Fill your shopping basket with fresh, in season fruits and vegetables, as they are rich sources of vitamins and minerals as well as fiber. Canned fruits and vegetables are good substitutes when the fresh varieties are out of season.

When choosing baked goods, always try to find those made with more nutritious and fiber rich whole wheat flour, wheat bran, oat bran, poppy seeds, sesame seeds, oatmeal or raisins.

Become a label reader. The federally mandated nutritional labels contain a wealth of valuable information for those who take the time to understand them. Nutritional labels contain valuable information on the calorie content, fiber content, and vitamin content of all packaged foods, and many meats, seafood and poultry products as well.

Finally, there are some popular myths about fiber. It is important to dispel these myths as you seek to increase the level of fiber in the diet.

The first myth concerns the relationship of crispness to level of fiber. In short, the crispness of a food is no indication of the amount of fiber it contains. For instance, the vegetables commonly used in salads, although crisp, are not significant sources of fiber. The crunch of the lettuce is a result of the amount of water it contains, not its fiber content.

Many people also think that cooking foods breaks down fiber – it does not. Cooking has no effect on the fiber content of foods. Peeling vegetables and fruits, however, does remove some of the fiber, since the skins of fruits and vegetables contain fiber. Edible skins, such as apple peels, can be good sources of fiber.

No matter what your reasons for increasing the amount of fiber in your diet, you may well find that this is one of the most positive dietary changes you ever make. Increasing fiber can have a significant impact on your future health and well being, and the change is easier to make than many people think.

27- Using fish as part of a healthy eating plan

It is hard to beat fish and seafood for high protein and low fat. Fish has been shown in study after study to have a positive impact on health, and to lower the risk of heart disease and other diseases. In addition, fish is delicious and easy to prepare.

Many nutrition experts recommend eating fish at least once or twice every week. The most nutritious varieties of fish, and those that contain the greatest amounts of heart protecting omega-3 fatty acids, tend to be those that live in cold ocean waters. These varieties of fish include salmon and sardines.

The benefits of a fishy diet

Fish has long been thought to have a positive benefit on the heart. So far the results of clinical studies have been inconclusive, but research into the heart healthy effects of fish continues. No matter what the benefits, there is little doubt that fish is a healthy food, containing significant levels of protein and smaller amounts of fat and calories than other types of meat.

As a matter of fact, fish is one of the best sources of protein there is. Everyone needs protein for building muscles and repairing damaged body tissues. In addition, protein plays a vital role in the growth of nails and hair, in hormone production and in many other vital bodily processes.

In addition to fish, many other animal based products, such as meat, eggs, poultry and dairy products, contain significant amounts of protein. Plant based sources of protein exist as well, in nuts, beans and lentils, among others.

The key to getting sufficient protein in the diet is to balance the healthy effects of protein on the diet against the large amounts of fat and cholesterol that protein rich foods often contain. The combination of high protein and low fat is one of the things that makes a diet rich in fish so appealing.

With the exception of salmon, almost all commonly eaten varieties of fish are very low in fat, and even salmon contains lower levels of fat than many varieties of meats. In addition, fish is low in saturated fat, the type of fat that is most associated with heart disease and clogged arteries.

Fish is low in unsaturated fat because of the nature of where and how they live. Instead of storing energy in the form of saturated fat as land animals do, fish store their fat in the form of polyunsaturated oils. That adaptation allows their bodies to function normally in the cool oceans and streams where they swim. It also makes them a great choice for anyone seeking to cut levels of saturated fat in the diet.

For all these reasons, fish remains an important part of any low fat, heart healthy lifestyle. Substituting high fat, greasy foods like hamburgers and ribs is a great way to make a change for healthy living.

One note about fish and pollution, however. It is true that many fish caught in polluted waters contain high levels of mercury. While most commercially caught and grown fish is low in mercury, it is important for fisherman to limit their consumption of locally caught fish. Pregnant women are also advised to limit their intake of fish, due to the potential harm to the baby.

Fitting fish into your busy lifestyle

Many people avoid fish because they do not know how to prepare and cook it. While it is true that fish can present more of a challenge for the inexperienced, there are many recipes and cookbooks that make preparation easier. In addition, many packaged seafood products contain cooking tips and serving suggestions that take some of the mystery out of preparing a nutritious and delicious meal of fresh fish.

Even those who do not cook, however, can enjoy the many benefits of fish in the diet. There are a number of canned seafood products on the market, including canned salmon, sardines and the ever popular tuna. So there is no reason fish cannot fit into your healthy eating plan.

28- Eat healthier by eating more fruits and vegetables

Recent changes in food guidelines have meant an increase in the recommended daily consumption of fruits and vegetables. That is because eating nutrient rich, low calorie, low fat foods such as fruits and vegetables, has been shown to have a strong impact on overall health.

In addition, high levels of fruits and vegetables in the diet has even been shown to help provide protection from a number of diseases and chronic conditions. There are ongoing studies on the relationship between a diet rich in fruits and vegetables and prevention of cancer, diabetes, heart disease and other conditions. While there may not yet be conclusive proof of a link between fruits and vegetables and lower risk of disease, there is ample anecdotal evidence to suggest that a healthy diet leads to a healthy body.

One reason for the strong health benefits of fruits and vegetables is their strong antioxidant qualities. Many fruits and vegetables are high in important antioxidant vitamins like vitamin C, vitamin E and vitamin A. In addition, fruits and vegetables contain lots of other nutrients and trace elements that are important to the proper function of the body.

Choosing the best fruits and vegetables is important, both to your health and the health of your food budget. We all have limited food budgets, and getting the best in terms of both taste and nutrition, is very important.

One way to get maximum value and maximum nutrition is to choose fresh, in season fruits and vegetables. That is because fresh, locally grown fruits and vegetables tend to be less expensive than their shipped counterparts.

If you have a farmers market or produce stand nearby, it can be an excellent source of the highest quality, lowest cost fruits and vegetables. Summer produce stands are excellent sources of delicious and nutritious fruits and vegetables.

In addition, buying fruits and vegetables as they come into season will instantly provide you with variety. There are literally hundreds of different varieties of fruits and vegetables at the average grocery store, and they all have different growing season. Buying the fresh in season fruits and vegetables is a great way to introduce yourself to some varieties you may never have tried before.

Of course there will be times when your favorite fruits and vegetables are not available locally. In those cases, frozen and canned varieties can do just fine. Just about every popular fruit and vegetable is available canned or frozen, and these can make wonderful, fast fruit salads or quick snacks.

It is important to choose fruits and vegetables in a variety of colors, and not only for ascetic reasons. Different colored fruits and vegetables contain different types of nutrients, and different levels of nutrients, so eating a good variety of green, gold, orange and purple is the best way to ensure adequate levels of nutrition.

How you cook the vegetables you buy is important as well. Over cooking can destroy many of the nutrients that make vegetables so healthy. Fortunately, most vegetables can be cooked by quickly steaming them in the microwave or on the stovetop.

How those cooked vegetables are served can also have a significant impact on their healthiness. Adding butter, margarine, oils or other fats to vegetables can quickly negate their health benefits. Better choices for seasoning cooked vegetables include fruit juices and low fat yogurt.

Most nutrition experts recommend that everyone eat from 5 to 9 servings of fruits or vegetables every day. While that may seem like an impossible goal, it is easier when you understand just what a serving consists of. One serving of a fruit or vegetable can be one medium sized piece of fruit, one slice of melon, two small pieces of fruit, one cup of strawberries, one cup of grapes, one half cup of canned fruit, one half cup of fruit salad, one side salad or one half cup of fresh fruit juice.

With all these choices to choose from, it is easy to see why fruits and vegetables are such a popular part of a healthy diet. No matter what your reason for pursuing healthy eating, fruits and vegetables are a healthy addition to any diet.

29- Eating healthy when money is tight

It is an unfortunate fact of life that many high nutrient, low fat, low calorie foods are expensive, while many nutrient free, calorie dense foods are cheap. This can make buying and cooking healthy foods for yourself and your family quite a challenge, particularly when the food budget is limited.

With some advance planning, however, it is still possible to create a week full of wonderful, nutritious meals, not matter how small your food budget. The key is to plan ahead, shop smart, and make the most out of the foods you buy.

Planning those meals

In today's busy world, meal planning often means calling out for a pizza or hitting the drive through on the way home. This type of lifestyle has helped to fuel the epidemic of obesity the country has been experiencing. There is a better way, however. Simply taking a few minutes a week to plan your family's meals can make a lot of difference, both in money saved and nutrition gained.

Advance meal planning is a must for any shopper on a budget. Writing down your meal plans, including the ingredients needed and expected preparation time, will help you plan what to buy and how to cook. For those with especially busy schedules, planning meals that can be cooked ahead of time and reheated is a huge time and money saver.

Fortunately, many healthy meals, such as vegetable casseroles, pasta dishes, meat dishes, seafood entrees, fruit salads, etc. are great as leftovers. It is easy to see how advance meal planning can save you time. Many working mothers, for instance, will make an entire week's worth of meals on the weekend, then heat each day's meals up as the week unfolds. This is a great strategy for creating a healthy and varied menu the whole family will love.

Hitting the grocery store

Now that you know what meals the coming week will bring, its time to hit the grocery store in search of the perfect and most healthy ingredients. Before you hit the grocery store, however, be sure to check the pantry. Keeping well stocked pantry, and restocking when staples such as canned vegetables and fruits go on sale, is the cornerstone of any healthy eating budget.

After you have gone through the pantry and noted the items you need to buy, it is time to check the sales flyers for your local grocery stores. Most major grocery store chains include sales flyers in the local newspaper, so be sure to check there for sales on the items you need for your meals.

Going to the grocery store armed with a shopping list is the best way to save both time and money. The grocery store contains many temptations, and most of them are both unhealthy and expensive. Sticking to the list is the best way to stay within your budget while providing yourself and your family with wholesome, nutritious food.

Don't forget to include fresh fruits and vegetables on your shopping list. Keeping fresh fruits and veggies around for snacks is a great way to eat healthier.

Preparing the meal

After everything has been purchased, the pantry has been restocked, and fresh bowls of fruits and vegetables are arranged for snacking, it is time to start creating that meal on a budget. As we said before, making meals in bulk for later use during the week is a great strategy for working women, and for those who are pressed for time. Taking a few hours to mix the ingredients and prepare the food can save a lot of time in the long run.

Of course for those on a budget saving money is just as important as saving time. One of the most important ways to save money while still eating a healthy diet is to stock up on those essentials you always seem to run out of. Try keeping a notepad on the refrigerator or near the sink. Every time you run out of a certain food, write it on the notepad. You will probably notice a pattern emerging after a week or two. So the next time your local grocery store runs a special on one of those things you always need, but it in bulk and keep a good supply on hand.

Buying in bulk is a great way to save money on many different kinds of healthy foods. Many people automatically think that the local warehouse club store is the cheapest place to buy bulk items, but this is not often the case. The weekly specials at the local grocery store often beat those warehouse club prices, often by a large margin. So be sure to shop around and comparison shop often as you put together those healthy meals.

30- Healthy eating without meat

As concerns about healthy eating have grown, so too has the interest in vegetarianism and veganism. Many nutrition experts recommend "eating low on the food chain". In plain language this means eating more grains, vegetables and fruits, and fewer meats, cheeses and other animal based products.

There are of course various levels of vegetarianism, and each type has its own unique health benefits and some health challenges as well. Of course vegetarians, like meat eaters, must still make healthy food choices. Simply pigging out on French fries while avoiding the burger will not make you a healthy vegetarian.

Some people who consider themselves vegetarians still eat poultry and seafood, while others avoid all animal flesh, even fish and chicken. Most vegetarians still eat milk, dairy products and eggs. In nutritional circles these people are referred to as lacto-ovo vegetarians.

Vegans, on the other hand, avoid all animal products, including eggs, milk and dairy products, and even fabrics like silk, leather and wool. It is vegans who face the largest challenges and risks when trying to follow a healthy diet. Most vegetarian diets provide more than enough nutrition, as long as smart dietary choices are made.

The key to eating a healthy vegetarian diet is much the same as eating a healthy diet that includes meat. It all boils down to making smart food choices, understanding nutritional labels, and cooking your vegetables to maximize their nutritional value.

Choosing the foods that make up the bulk of a vegetarian diet is very important. For most vegetarians, vegetables, grains, lentils and soy products will make up the bulk of their diet, and these staples are included in many vegetarian recipes.

When cooking with soy, however, it is important to remember that tofu is relatively high in fat. The fat content of tofu dishes is often comparable to that of dishes that are made with lean cuts of meat. Those vegetarians following a low fat diet may want to limit the amount of tofu based products they eat.

The same caution applies to the nuts and seeds that can make up a large part of a vegetarian diet. Nuts and seeds are excellent sources of dietary protein, but they can be high in fat as well.

Many newly minted vegetarians worry that they will not be able to get enough protein and iron without eating meat, but for most vegetarians this is not a problem. Most diets today actually contain too much protein, and there are many non animal derived sources of protein for vegetarians to enjoy.

Proper cooking techniques are of course very important to any healthy diet. Avoiding high fat cooking methods is important, as is avoiding the use of high fat creams, butters and sauces. A vegetable stir fry cooked in healthy olive oil can be a great addition to any vegetarian menu. And a great fruit salad is both easy to make and delicious as a snack or a meal.

The only real area of concern when it comes to vegetarianism and health is the B-complex vitamins, particularly vitamin B12. Vitamin B12 is almost exclusively derived from animal based sources, so vegans, who avoid all animal products, should take a high quality vitamin B12 or B-complex vitamin supplement. It is also important for vegans to discuss their diet and lifestyle with their family physicians. As vegetarianism and veganism becomes more widespread, the amount of information on the nutritional needs of these two groups continues to grow.

The bottom line is that vegetarians can enjoy a very healthy lifestyle. Making vegetables, fruits, whole grains and beans the centerpiece of the diet is a smart move for many people, and a good low fat vegetarian diet can be a great way to enjoy a healthy lifestyle. As with a meat based diet, however, it is important for vegetarians to follow common sense eating guidelines and make smart choices when creating meat free meals.

31- Smart shopping tips for healthy eating

Any healthy eating plan begins at the grocery store. Learning to make smart choices when shopping for food is the key to the success of any healthy diet plan. Learning to recognize the healthiest, freshest foods is a skill every grocery shopper must learn.

Of course, the logical place to start the healthy shopping trip to the grocery store is at the produce section. Most large modern supermarkets have huge produce sections, often taking up a large portion of the store. It is not unusual for the produce section alone to contain hundreds of choices, so it can be difficult to know the best foods to choose.

When it comes to the produce section of the supermarket, however, it is difficult to make a bad choice. That is because almost all fruits and vegetables are healthy, low in calories and delicious. While there are some high fat fruits and vegetables, such as avocados, they are the exception rather than the rule.

The most important thing to remember when shopping for fruits and vegetables is the old saw that variety is the spice of life. Trying a variety of different fruits and vegetables, including some you may never have heard of before.

Eating a wide variety of fruits and vegetables is a great way to enjoy a healthier diet without becoming bored. Many new diets fail due to boredom, but eating a large number of different fruits and vegetables every day can virtually eliminate that problem.

One way to introduce this variety into a healthy diet is to seek out fresh, in season produce on every trip to the grocery store. Not only are fresh, locally grown fruits and vegetables usually less expensive, but the changing variety will help guarantee fresh new recipes week after week.

Of course the produce section is not the only place to find healthy, nutritious foods. The other parts of the supermarket are also full of both good and bad choices. For instance, when choosing bread, it is best to buy whole grain breads and avoid the more processed varieties. The same is true of baked goods. Whole grain products contain large amounts of fiber and other nutrients that the more refined baked goods may lack.

Important healthy eating decisions need to be made in the meat section of the grocery store as well. This means buying the leanest cuts of meat you can find. In addition, extra fat should be trimmed from the edges of steaks, roasts and chops. You can do this trimming at home, or, better yet, have the butcher do it at the store. After all, why pay extra for what you won't use?

Even though poultry is generally low fat, not all poultry is created equal. Some varieties, like duck and goose, contain significant amounts of fat. A roast goose or duck can be great for Christmas or other special occasions, but these meats are generally too greasy to be used for everyday meals.

Even low fat poultry like chicken breasts can benefit from some additional trimming. Removing the skin from chicken significantly cuts the amount of fat and calories it contains. In addition, using low fat white meat chicken instead of fattier dark meat is a smart move.

When buying ground meats, always try to buy the leanest varieties you can afford. Ground beef that is 97% lean is a good choice. In addition, ground turkey or ground chicken makes a good, lower fat substitute for ground beef, and it can be used in all recipes that call for ground beef, including tacos, burritos, barbeque, burgers, etc.

One important note about ground turkey and ground chicken, however. Processed ground poultry products can often contain surprisingly high levels of fat. That is because manufacturers often grind up unwanted skin and fat in addition to the lean turkey or chicken. This is a particular problem with lower priced varieties of ground chicken and turkey, so it pays to read the labels and monitor fat content carefully.

Learning to be a smart shopper is a vital part of enjoying a healthy lifestyle.. No matter what your reason for eating healthy, learning to shop smart and buy healthy foods is an essential first step.

32- Choosing the leanest cuts of meat for healthy eating

Choosing the right cuts of meat is one of the most difficult things to do when following a healthy lifestyle. Meat can be among the most calorie and fat dense foods, and it is not always easy to spot the leanest cuts of meat in the butcher's case.

It is important, however, to choose lean cuts of meat when cooking healthy dishes. Even the lowest fat meal can be sabotaged by the addition of a high fat pork chop, roast or other cut of meat.

Of course it is still possible to include meat in a healthy diet. There are many lean cuts of meat available at the local grocery store, and meet provides much needed protein for energy and muscle development.

The key to buying the leanest cuts of meat for your healthy diet is to examine the cuts of meat carefully, and to have any additional fat trimmed. In cases where the grocery store has its own butcher, this is a relatively easy process. Most in store butchers are happy to show customers the various cuts of meat, and to trip the meat to their specification.

In the case of grocery stores where all the cuts of meat is prepackaged, choosing the leanest cuts is often more difficult. Meat is often packaged to conceal the fat, so additional trimming may need to be done once the meat is purchased.

It is important, however, to trim meat carefully, no matter where it is purchased. Trimming the extra fat off the meat you cook is very important when preparing healthy meals for yourself and your family.

Shopping for good cuts of poultry is much easier than finding the leanest cuts of meat. That is because the most common poultry products, such as chicken and turkey, are naturally low fat. There are high fat varieties of poultry, such as goose and duck, but these are not served on a regular basis in most homes.

The biggest problem poultry shoppers face is the calories and fat added by chicken and turkey skin. Most grocery stores sell skinless varieties of chicken breast, and these can be a great time saver. If the skinless varieties are a lot more expensive, however, it may be more cost effective to buy the cheaper cuts and remove the skin yourself.

Like poultry, most varieties of seafood are naturally low in fat. Salmon is probably the best known exception to this rule; salmon is fatty for fish, but still much leaner than many cuts of meat. Most varieties of fish, however, are naturally lean and very healthy.

As a matter of fact, those striving to follow a healthy diet should try to add more fish and seafood to their diet. Fish is very high in protein, and low in fat and relatively low in calories. This is a valuable combination for any one food.

As with many aspects of smart food shopping, when it comes to meat, poultry and seafood, fresher is better. There are a number of prepackaged, ready to heat and eat, varieties of meat, seafood and chicken at the local grocery store. While these products can be fine for an occasional quick meal or snack, they should not form the basis of a healthy diet.

The reason for this is simple. Processing meats, seafood and poultry often involves the use of unhealthy additives such as preservatives and sodium. Check the sodium level of any processed meat products you buy, and use such products only occasionally.

While buying fresh meat, seafood and poultry products is best, it is important to handle such foods properly on their journey from the grocery store to the dinner table. Improper food handling is responsible for the vast majority of food borne illness in the United States, and it is important to handle any raw meat, seafood or poultry product carefully.

Probably the most important part of food handling safety is making sure that foods that are not cooked, such as salads and breads, do not come into contact with raw meat, poultry or seafood. Most food borne pathogens are killed during the cooking process, but they can easily spread to salads and other uncooked foods if care is not used.

That means scrubbing counter tops carefully with an antibacterial product, using separate cutting boards for meats and vegetables, and of course washing your hands thoroughly after handling meat, poultry or seafood products.

33- Healthier low fat eating

Avoiding high levels of fat is important to just about everyone these days. High levels of dietary fat and cholesterol have been implicated in heart disease, stroke, diabetes, and even some types of cancers. Staying healthy often means cutting back on fat. The trick is to do this without sacrificing the taste you and your family crave.

There are many good reasons for cutting back on the amount of fat in the diet. The average diet today contains far too much fat, and lowering the level of fat in the diet is a great help for losing weight and gaining fitness. Since fat contains more than twice as many calories as protein or carbohydrates, cutting back on fat usually means a reduction in caloric intake.

In addition to its usefulness in losing weight, cutting levels of fat in the diet is also important to long term good health. High fat in the diet can lead to high cholesterol levels, hardening of the arteries, obesity, diabetes and other serious medical complications. In addition, high dietary fat is though to play a role in the development of some of the most common cancers.

In addition, cutting back on high fat foods will allow you to enjoy more of other, healthier foods. Enjoying more wholesome, healthy foods like vegetables, fruits and whole grains while cutting back on greasy, fatty foods, is a great way to enjoy a healthy lifestyle.

Cutting back on the amount of fat in the diet is not always easy, however, especially for those who have never had to worry about fat content before. There are a number of simple, easy changes you can make, however, that will allow you to enjoy a low fat lifestyle with little sacrifice.

For instance, when enjoying toast, bagels and other whole grain products, don't use peanut butter or cream cheese, which are high in fat. For a low fat alternative, spread toast, bread and bagels with jelly, jams, apple butter, low fat cream cheese or low fat margarine.

Eating a healthier, lower fat diet often means changing your relationship with high fat foods. That means enjoying high fat foods like bacon and sausage as an occasional treat or garnish, instead of as a staple of the diet.

Eating healthy naturally means eating more salads, but it is important not to wreck the healthy effects of the salad by loading them down with high fat dressings. A salad tricked out with blue cheese dressing, for instance, can easily contain more fat and calories than a hamburger. That is why it is important to keep a supply of low fat or nonfat dressings on hand. When eating at your favorite restaurant, ask for nonfat dressing, or get the dressing on the side so you can control the amount used.

Baked potatoes are another healthy alternative, but like salads, they can be sabotaged by the addition of high fat dressings. Instead of using butter, margarine, cheese or sour cream, try topping baked potatoes with plain nonfat yogurt, salsa, cottage cheese or steamed broccoli. And don't forget to eat the potato skin for extra nutrients. The skins of baked potatoes are great sources of fiber and vitamins.

When using seasonings, there are a number of great garnishes that add zest and flavor without adding calories. Additions like lemon juice, salsa, herbs and green onions are great additions to salads and stir fried vegetables.

You're probably seeing a pattern here. Toppings can be great when used wisely, but the wrong toppings can quickly add fat and calories to even the lowest fat recipe. Use high fat toppings sparingly, and try to find low fat and nonfat alternatives whenever possible.

There are a great many low fat and nonfat products on the market, and these products make it easier than ever to eat healthy while still enjoying your favorite foods. Some of the best low fat and nonfat foods are found in the dairy case, including low fat and nonfat milk, cheese and even ice cream.

Many popular snacks, including cakes, cookies and even potato chips, are available in nonfat and low fat varieties as well. Care should be used, however, with such products. Some of these baked goods and salty snacks have very high levels of sugar, sweeteners, salt and other unhealthy ingredients. As with all snacks, low fat cakes, cookies and chips should be an occasional treat only. Instead, snack on fresh fruit like apples, oranges and bananas.

34- Living and eating for maximum nutrition

The past few years have seen a bit of a resurgence of interest in healthy living and healthy eating, and that is a good thing. We all know that most people do not eat enough fruits and vegetables, and that many people eat too much of the wrong things – like sugar, salt and fat. Reversing this trend will take some time and some effort, but starting with your own diet is a great way to improve your health and your life.

The key to changing your diet, of course, is to change it is ways that you can live with for a lifetime. The reason that most diet and lifestyle changes fail is that they are too difficult to follow once the initial excitement has worn off. The key is to make small changes, simple changes, that you can follow for the rest of your life.

Where you start your healthy eating plan depends in great part on your particular goals. For many people, a healthy eating program can be as simple as eating more fruits and vegetables. For others, a healthy eating plan will require a radical change in the way they shop, cook, and eat.

Since healthy eating means so many different things to different people, it is impossible to come up with a single healthy eating guide that will be right for everyone. The runner toning up for a marathon will have different nutritional needs than the factor worker who wants to lose 20 pounds.

No matter what the goal, however, it is important to eat a variety of foods, and to make smart choices when shopping, when cooking and when eating. Eating out can present special challenges, and it is important to familiarize yourself with the ingredients of the foods you order in your favorite restaurant.

Making healthy food choices means eating more of the good foods – like vegetables, fruits, whole grains, etc., and less of the bad foods, like salt, sugar and fats.

Starting by eating more high nutrition, low calorie foods is a good place to start. Luckily, the produce section of the local grocery store likely contains hundreds of different examples of such foods. Fruits and vegetables are almost always low in calories and fat, and they are generally very nutritious as well.

Since variety is so important to a healthy diet, it is a good idea to try out a sampling of different fruits and vegetables on your first healthy eating shopping trip. Start with some of the fruits and vegetables you have always wanted to try but never gotten around to. For instance, many people have never tasted asparagus, spinach or Brussels sprouts. While some love these foods and others hate them, you will never know unless you try them for yourself.

This kind of foraging is a great way to introduce yourself to foods you have never tried before. It is a great way to try new things, and you just might discover a new favorite food while you're at it.

Experimenting with cooking all these exotic fruits and vegetables is another great idea. There are a ton of healthy cooking recipes and cookbooks on the market, and a new cookbook can be a great motivator for healthy eating.

It is important to remember that making your diet healthier does not necessarily mean making a radical change. Simple changes, like trimming the excess fat off of a steak, or substituting nonfat yogurt for sour cream on your baked potato, can go a long way toward enjoying a healthier lifestyle.

As a matter of fact, in the long run the simplest and easiest to follow changes are the ones that matter most. That is because making easy changes means that you will be able to stick with them for the long run. Healthy eating is a marathon, not a sprint.

32- The five a day rule and healthier eating

If you have not heard of the five a day rule before, that is about to change. The five a day rule refers to the recommended daily servings of fruits and vegetables. Health experts recommend that every eat – yes you guessed it – five a day.

That five a day guideline is actually the minimum recommendation, and eating up to nine servings a day of fruits and vegetables is a great way to increase health, lower dietary fat, increase vitamin consumption and just generally feel better.

Following the five a day rule may just be the most important, and one of the easiest, changes you can make in your daily diet. There are many reasons to increase your consumption of fruits and vegetables, including:

> ➤ They are delicious
> ➤ They are nutritious

> ➤ They are colorful
> ➤ They are plentiful
> ➤ They are inexpensive

It is hard to find such a great combination in any other food group. Delicious, nutritious and affordable foods can be hard to find, but they abound in the produce section of virtually any grocery store.

In order to make fruits and vegetables even more affordable, it is best to buy them when they are in season. Every type of fruit and vegetable grown in this country has its own growing season, and fruits and vegetables that are out of season usually must be purchased in frozen, dried or canned varieties.

Fresh, in season, fruits and vegetables, on the other hand, are usually plentiful and inexpensive. And in addition to the grocery store, such produce is often available at farmers markets and even at roadside stands. This locally grown produce is often of superior quality and lower price than that at the supermarket, so if you have such a venue in your area by all means check it out.

It has long been known that fruits and vegetables play an important role in a healthy diet, and science continues to confirm this fact with study after study. Diets high in fruits and vegetables and low in fats have been shown to play a role in preventing infections, protecting the heart and even in protecting against some kinds of cancer.

One reason for this is that many fruits and vegetables are rich in antioxidants. Antioxidants are able to protect the body from damage by free radicals. Free radicals are naturally occurring compounds thought to play a role in many diseases.

One quick and easy way to take care of one fifth of the five a day rule is to start every day with a fresh glass of fruit juice. Apple juice, orange juice and grapefruit juice are all excellent choices. When choosing juice, however, be sure that it is 100% real fruit juice and not a blend. Fruit juice blends can contain high levels of sugar and low levels of fruit.

A quick fruit salad is another excellent way to satisfy part of the five a day rule. It is easy to make a quick fruit salad using either canned or fresh fruits. In addition, canned fruit salads are widely available and often a great value. As with juice, however, it is important to read the label and be sure that there is no added sugar. Fruit is sweet enough on its own – extra sugar is something you simply do not need.

Another interesting way to increase fruit and vegetable consumption is to use them as garnishes for other foods. For instance, adding strawberries, blueberries or bananas to your morning cereal is a great way to increase the flavor of the cereal while at the same time increasing the amount of fruit in your diet.

And adding vegetables like green peppers, red peppers and chunks of pineapples to shish kebobs is a great way to grill your way to good health. Your kebobs will be more colorful, more attractive, and of course more healthy.

No matter how you choose to meet the five a day rule, there is no doubt that increasing the amount of fruits and vegetables in the diet can have a profound effect on health. Many who have eaten more fruits and vegetables report greater levels of energy, a greater sense of well being, fewer colds and more stamina. So why not follow the simple five a day plan to good health?

Eat Healthier: Tips for healthy eating

33- Enjoy healthy eating with citrus fruits

There are few single food groups with as much to recommend them, and as many health benefits, as citrus fruits. Citrus fruits are packed full of a number of important vitamins and minerals, as well as fiber. In addition, citrus fruits are delicious, abundant, and usually quiet inexpensive.

Citrus fruits abound in most modern grocery stores, even in the winter months. Thanks to modern distribution networks, citrus fruits grown around the world are easily accessible in the supermarkets of this country.

Of course many people prefer locally grown citrus fruits, but when they are not available, shipped citrus is a good substitute. There is a growing season for each kind of citrus in various parts of the country, so it pays to familiarize yourself with those seasons in order to take advantage of the freshest locally grown tomatoes, oranges, grapefruits and more.

Citrus fruits are perfect for anytime of day, from a grapefruit in the morning to an orange at lunchtime to a dinner salad piled high with locally grown tomatoes.

Citrus fruits contain so many important vitamins and minerals that it would be impossible to list them all. Citrus fruits are a good example of why fresh fruits and vegetables are a better source of complete nutrition than vitamin supplements. While some of the important vitamins and nutrients contained in citrus fruits have been identified and synthesized, others, particularly the many trace minerals, have not. There is simply no pharmacological substitute for healthy eating.

Vitamin C is probably the most important, and the most well known, nutrient provided by citrus fruits like oranges and grapefruits. Vitamin C has been widely studied, and it is thought to play an important role in keeping us healthy.

Vitamin C plays a vital role in keeping skin and gums healthy, and in protecting the cells of the body from damage by free radicals. And since vitamin C is a water soluble vitamin, it is important to eat foods high in vitamin C every day. Vitamin C is not stored in the body like fat soluble vitamins are, and any vitamin C not used each day is excreted.

Fortunately, it is easy to get the vitamin C you need each day from citrus fruits. For instance, a single orange contains over 150% percent of the RDA (recommended daily allowance) of vitamin C.

Many people do not realize, that in addition to vitamin C, oranges, grapefruits and other citrus fruits also contain significant amounts of fiber. Fiber plays an important role in digestion, and it is thought to have protective qualities against heart disease and some forms of cancer. In addition, fiber is thought to have the ability to lower high levels of cholesterol in the blood.

Perhaps the most important benefit of citrus fruits is the presence of folic acid. This important vitamin is known to prevent many neural cord birth defects such as spina bifida when consumed early in a pregnancy, and for this reason folic acid has been added to everything from bread to cereal. It is best, however for women and men alike to get this important nutrient from the foods they eat, and citrus fruits are rich in folic acid.

Potassium is another important benefit of citrus fruits. When many people think of potassium, they think of bananas, but bananas are not the only fruit that contains significant levels of potassium. Many citrus fruits also contain plenty of potassium.

Potassium levels are very important to good health, since potassium plays a role in maintaining proper levels of bodily fluids, and it also affects the absorption of other nutrients. The stresses of modern life, including consumption of caffeine and alcohol, stress and dehydration, can all play havoc with potassium levels, so it is important to eat foods rich in potassium every day.

With all these advantages, it is easy to see why citrus fruits are so popular. Even people who do not normally eat fruits and vegetables often have a hard time saying no to a great glass of orange juice or a nice juicy grapefruit.

34- The importance of high fiber low fat foods

One of the easiest and most effective changes you can make to your diet is to eat more foods rich in fiber, and fewer foods rich in fat. There are many reasons to boost the intake of fiber while controlling fat, including increased fitness, decreased weight and better overall health.

It is a fact that most people consume too much of what they should not – things like sugar, salt and fat, and not enough of what they should – like vegetables, fruits, and whole grains. That means that many people are not getting sufficient fiber in their diets, and they may suffer a variety of heath effects as a result.

Of course before you can eat more fiber you need to know where that fiber comes from. Gauging the amount of fiber in your diet is yet another reason to read nutritional labels carefully. All packaged and processed foods in the grocery store must carry these labels, and they detail such things as fat, fiber, calories and nutrient values. Getting familiar with these nutritional labels is a necessary first step to improving any diet.

One important note about increasing the level of fiber in your diet. While increasing fiber and decreasing fat is certainly a worthy goal, it is best to take things gradually until your body adjusts to the change. Those accustomed to low levels of fiber often experience bloating, cramps, gas and abdominal pain when suddenly boosting the amount of fiber in their diet. Increasing the level of fiber gradually helps to avoid these unpleasant side effects.

Most plant based foods contain at least some fiber, but some types of foods contain more than others. The only foods that do not contain fiber are animal based products. That means that meats, poultry, seafood, eggs, milk and dairy products do not contain any fiber. It is important to keep that fact in mind when planning healthy meals.

The foods highest in fiber, containing more than 6 grams per serving, include such healthy staples as dried beans, legumes, dried peas, dried fruits, nuts, sunflower seeds, sesame seeds and many types of berries. These foods are excellent sources of fiber.

Not as high in fiber as those above, but still great sources of fiber are apples, pears, barley, bran muffins, lima beans, brown rice, snow peas, green peas and sweet potatoes. Baked potatoes are also good sources of fiber, as long as the skin is consumed along with the flesh of the potato. All these foods contain from 4 to 6 grams of fiber per serving.

Many vegetables and fruits also contain fiber, as does rye bread, wheat bead and melons. Most of these foods contain from 2 to 4 grams of fiber, so you will need to add more of them to get the most out of their fiber content.

It is important to take fiber content into account as you do your weekly grocery shopping. Getting into the habit of reading labels and choosing high fiber foods is the best way to make a long term commitment to healthier eating.

It is important to choose foods high in fiber during every trip to the grocery store. When choosing bread, crackers and other baked goods, for instance, you should strive to find whole grain varieties that are rich in fiber. Wheat and rye bread are good sources of fiber, as are bran muffins and many kinds of cereal.

Choosing cereals that are rich in fiber is a great way to increase the level of fiber intake while enjoying a delicious breakfast every morning. Cereals that contain wheat bran and oat bran can be excellent sources of fiber. The most important thing is to read the nutritional label and not rely simply on the claims made on the box.

Many people are under the assumption that cooking fresh vegetables and other fiber rich foods destroys their fiber content, but luckily this is not the case. While it is true that overcooking certain vegetables can result in some loss of nutrients, cooking has no effect whatsoever on fiber content. So feel free to prepare those healthy foods any way you want.

35- Making fish and seafood part of a healthy diet

Maximizing protein content while minimizing fat and calories is a goal of many people who are trying to lose weight, gain fitness or just enjoy a healthier diet. There are few foods that combine low fat, low calories and high protein the way fish and seafood do.

In addition, the protective oils in many cold water fish are being studied for their possible role in preventing heart disease and lowering levels of cholesterol in the bloods.

In addition, fish dishes are delicious, easy to prepare and often inexpensive. Many people have avoided buying more fish because they were unsure of how to cook and prepare it. While fish dishes can sometimes be a challenge, there are many recipes, both online and in cookbooks, that make it easier than ever to prepare fresh fish for yourself and your family.

Many nutritionists recommend that everyone eat fish at least twice a week.

Substituting low fat, low calorie fish dishes for more calorie dense, fatty meats is a great way to lower the amount of total fat in your diet, and this can boost your level of fitness or help you lose weight.

The amount of protein in fresh and frozen fish and seafood is very high, certainly comparable to higher fat sources like beef, pork and lamb. And fish is generally thought to be a healthier choice, since all that protein comes with less fat and fewer calories. Everyone knows about the importance of protein in the diet, for both children and adults. Protein is a vital building block of muscle, and it plays a role in repairing muscle damage, growing strong nails and hair and other important bodily functions.

While protein is found mainly in animal based foods such as meat, poultry, seafood, eggs and dairy products, there are plant based sources of protein as well. These non animal sources of protein include peanut butter, lentils, peas and nuts. The downside to many protein laden plant based foods, however is their high content.

This is yet another feature that makes fish so appealing as a source of protein. Fish contains just as much protein as many of these higher fat, higher calorie sources. Eating fish provides – shall we say – a greater protein bang for the buck than many other sources.

You may have heard that salmon contains a lot of fat, and it is true that salmon does contain more fat than many other fish. Compared to high fat meats like sausage and bacon, however, salmon is still a relatively low fat source of protein. Like other fatty foods, however, it is important for those watching their fat intake to limit their consumption of salmon.

One advantage fish has over other types of meats is the type of fat it contains. Most meats contain saturated fats, which are solid at room temperature. Unlike cattle, pigs and other land animals, the fat in fish is of the polyunsaturated variety. Polyunsaturated fats are liquid at room temperature, and they are healthier fats for the people who consume them.

Saturated fats are thought to play a greater role in heart disease, stroke and hardening of the arteries. That is why healthy cooking typically involves the use of polyunsaturated fats such as canola oil and olive oil, instead of saturated fats such as beef lard and butter.

Many people worry about the level of pollution in general, and mercury contamination in particular, in fish. While it is true that polluted waters are of some concern when it comes to fish, seafood products are actually quite safe to eat.

In addition, many types of fish, like salmon and sardines, are farm raised, and their diet and environment is strictly controlled. It is recommended, however, that fishermen and fisherwomen limit the amount of their catch that is eaten if they live near a polluted river or stream. The local fishing and hunting authority usually issues guidelines for eating fish in areas where pollution is a problem.

36- Enjoy a healthier lifestyle with more fruits and vegetables

Everyone agrees on the importance of eating more fruits and vegetables, but not enough people are following this important advice. Increasing your consumption of fruits and vegetables is one of the easiest changes you can make to increase your level of health, lose weight and gain fitness.

No matter what your reason for pursuing a healthier diet, eating more fruits and vegetables is a great way to enjoy a delicious varied diet while enjoying greater levels of health.

Everyone knows the importance of a healthy diet to a healthy body, and fruits and vegetables are rich in the vitamins, minerals, trace elements and other micronutrients that make a diet healthy.

In addition to all these advantages, fruits and vegetables are colorful, easy to use, abundant and inexpensive. Fruits and vegetables are great in soups, salads, as side dishes and as main courses. There are so many varieties of fruits and vegetables, and so many different ways to use them, that it is almost impossible to get bored with them.

One reason for the recommendation that everyone increase their consumption of fruits and vegetables is that many of these foods have been shown to have strong antioxidant qualities. Antioxidants are important to good health due to their ability to bind with and neutralize harmful elements called free radicals. These free radicals are thought to play a role in cancer, aging related illnesses and other conditions.

Normally, free radicals are neutralized automatically as part of the body's natural processes. However, when the immune system has been weakened, or if you are just feeling run down, these antioxidant fighters may not be working at peak efficiency. Many fruits and vegetables have high amounts of many antioxidant vitamins, including vitamin A, vitamin E and vitamin C.

Since there are so many fruits and vegetables to choose from, it is important to choose the best ones for your diet. Of courses, the perfect fruits and vegetables for you are the ones you like the best. After all, you will have a hard time taking advantage of all that nutrition unless you actually eat the fruits and vegetables you buy.

Getting the most fruits and vegetables for your limited food budget is an important consideration for most people. Fruits and vegetables are usually plentiful and inexpensive, but in some cases they can be somewhat pricey, especially in the winter months when most fruits and vegetables must be shipped long distances.

In addition to the supermarket and local grocery store, farmers markets can be places to find the freshest fruits and vegetables at the lowest possible prices. Farmers markets and roadside produce stands are often excellent sources of fresh, high quality fruits and vegetables.

Even when there is no farmers market nearby, it is still possible to get great, high quality fruits and vegetables at some excellent prices, simply by buying those fruits and vegetables as they come into season. Buying in season fruits and vegetables is usually cheaper than buying produce that comes from far away, and locally grown produce is often fresher and more nutritious as well.

Many people recommend buying a variety of colors when shopping for fruits and vegetables, and not just because they look good on the plate together. Different colored fruits and vegetables have different nutritional qualities, so eating a wide variety of colors will give you the best selection of flavors, textures, tastes and nutrients.

Cooking vegetables properly is important as well, since overcooking can destroy some of the nutritional value of many vegetables. Green leafy vegetables such as spinach, kale, broccoli and Brussels sprouts are particularly vulnerable to nutrient loss due to overcooking.

It is best to lightly steam vegetables in the microwave on the top of the stove. When steaming vegetables for maximum nutrition, it is important to use as little water as possible. Use only enough water to keep the vegetable from burning, and remove them from the heat source as soon as possible.

No matter what your reason for following a healthy diet, we believe you will find that eating more fruits and vegetables is a delicious, as well as a nutritious, way to get the vitamins and minerals you need every day.

37- How to cook for a healthier you

When it comes to healthy eating, sometimes how you cook is just as important as what you eat. There are definitely healthy, and less healthy, ways to prepare the healthy foods you buy.

When it comes to cooking vegetables, it is always best to use as little water as possible. That is because over cooking, especially when boiling, can destroy some of the important nutrients that make vegetables so important.

The best way to cook most vegetables in the microwave, preferably in a special microwave vegetable steamer. Vegetables can also be lightly cooked in a microwave safe bowl, using as little water as possible.

Vegetables can be cooked on the stove top as well, but it is important to use as little water as possible when boiling vegetables. Vegetables like broccoli and Brussels sprouts are particularly susceptible to losing important nutrients.

Microwave ovens are also great for making other vegetables, especially baked potatoes. Baked potatoes get great in the microwave, with the skins getting nice and crispy and the flesh being very tender. Of course this means that less high fat toppings may be needed, so the microwave is a great way to make nutritious and delicious baked potatoes.

Grilling is another great way to make healthy, delicious meals. Grilling meats is a great, low fat way to prepare meats, and it is a great way to make vegetables and fruits as well. Vegetable kebobs are great on the grill, whether combined with lean cuts of meat or made into a meal of their own.

Your oven's broiler is another great way to create low fat meals. Broiling is a great way to prepare all kinds of meats and seafood, and broiling is a low fat cooking method as well. Broiling fish is a great, fast and easy way to prepare this staple of a healthy low fat diet, while broiling steaks and chops keep fat at a minimum while keeping taste at its highest.

The handy kitchen blender is another great way to create delicious snacks using healthy fruits and vegetables. Blenders are great for making fruit smoothies, and most recipes call for little more than crushed ice, fruit juice and fresh fruit.

Some great, high nutrition, low fat, low calorie meals require no preparation at all. For instance, it is possible to make a wonderful, and easy, fruit salad with just a can of mandarin oranges, an apple, some strawberries and a banana. Simply open the can of mandarin oranges, empty it into a bowl, along with the juice it is packed in. Then add banana slices, apples slices and strawberries. For extra color and taste, add some blueberries, raspberries or raisins. The total prep time for this great creation is all of five minutes.

Fruit skewers are another creative, healthy and easy meal or snack. Simply take shish kebob skewers and stack them full of melon slices, strawberries, red grapes, white grapes and chunks of pineapple. Plain nonfat yogurt makes an excellent and low fat dip.

In addition to the above ideas, making your own homemade salsa is a great way to create a low fat alternative to sour cream and other high fat dips. Salsa can be made using healthy ingredients like tomatoes, mangoes, avocados, onions, cilantro and lime juice.

In addition, perking up a plain salad is a great way to add even more fruits and vegetables to an already healthy diet. For example, use broccoli florets, carrot slices, slices of cucumber, green peppers, red peppers, and bean sprouts to add color, zest and flavor to any salad.

Cucumbers, green peppers, broccoli and carrots are also great additions to pasta salads and potato salads. Adding extra crunch and color is a great way to add zest to any meal or snack.

Even a plain green salad of lettuce and tomatoes can be enhanced through the use of colorful fruits and vegetables. Adding vegetables like carrots, bean sprouts, and spinach leaves, and fruits like mandarin oranges, apple slices, nectarine slices, grapes, apple slices, pineapples and raisins, adds both beauty and taste to any salad.

Of course salad dressing is always an important subject for those trying to follow a healthy lifestyle. High fat dressing can sabotage even the healthiest salad, but there are many excellent, low fat and healthy choices when it comes to topping a salad. Using flavored vinegars, herbs and fruit juices are novel approaches to salad dressing, in addition to the many nonfat and low fat versions of commercial salad dressing.

38- Healthy cooking for those with little time

Everyone who has ever juggled home, family and kids knows how difficult it is to create healthy meals when pressed for time. Cooking healthy, delicious meals can be difficult, but some advance planning can allow you to make the most of your cooking time.

One way to cook healthy meals that are easy to prepare is to plan your meals around several key foods that can be prepared in large quantities and used in several different recipes on consecutive nights. This method of making meals last is totally different from the usual strategy of making a huge batch of food and living on leftovers for the rest of the week. Your family will certainly appreciate the difference.

There are some key elements to cooking this way. The first step is to promptly separate and refrigerate the portion that will be used for the next days meal before you place tonight's meal on the table. Refrigerating the unused portion of the prepared meal is important to preventing food borne illnesses, especially when serving meat, poultry, seafood or any meal containing eggs or dairy products.

The foods that have been prepared ahead of time should be stored in shallow containers to allow it to cool more quickly in the refrigerator. Thicker foods like stews, puddings and meat slices should be stored in bowls no deeper than two inches. The food should be stirred occasionally as it cools.

The left over refrigerated foods should be used within one to two days. If the food is to be stored longer than that, it should be frozen for later use and thawed overnight in the refrigerator. Thawing food at room temperature should be avoided, since it can be a gateway to food borne illnesses and other pathogens.

One of the easiest examples of the leftover strategy is chicken breasts or turkey cutlets. Poultry works great for this strategy, since it is easy to cook large quantities.

Start by cooking extra chicken breasts or turkey cutlets. Half of the chicken or turkey should be refrigerated overnight for use the next day. The remaining half can be topped with your favorite spices, sauces and seasonings and served right away.

The brilliance of this strategy will become apparent the next evening, when the other half of the turkey or chicken can be used in an entirely different way. One great way to use the other half is to cut it into strips, add lettuce and salad dressing and create a delicious Caesar salad. Thus one staple food becomes two delicious and totally different meals.

Rice is another great staple that works well for planned ahead meals. The rice dishes start with cooking and preparing a large quantity of rice. While the rice is cooking, add some ground beef or ground turkey to tomato sauce and flavor it with some Italian seasonings. Pour it over the rice and serve your family a great meal.

On the second night, take the remaining rice, fry it in a skillet and mix it will your favorite vegetables and perhaps a can of shrimp or crab for another, totally different rice based meal.

The leftover rice can also be saved and combined with turkey, chicken or beef from previous meals to create different flavor combinations, including casseroles and soups.

Rice makes a great staple for nay meal preparation plan. In addition to its versatility, rice is also easy to freeze. After the cooked rice has been cooled in the fridge, it is easy to transfer to freezer bags and saved for future quick, easy and healthy meals.

No matter how short of time you are, it is still possible to create delicious, nutritious meals in no time. Making a week's worth of meals in only a few hours will give you more time to enjoy your food and your family.

39- Healthy snacks for healthy living

Snacking is one of those issues that can wreck the best laid plan for healthier eating. Everyone wants a snack now and then, but the key is to make those snacks healthy and nutritious as well as delicious.

There are many great snacks that can be enjoyed guilt free. For instance choosing snacks from whole grain products, fruits and vegetables, milk and dairy products, meat and nuts can be a great way to satisfy your craving without destroying your diet.

The world of grain and whole grain products contain a great many healthy snacks, including whole grain breads (wheat bread and rye bread are great choices), whole what bagels, wholesome tortilla shells, pita bread and whole grain cereals.

The all important vegetable and fruit food group contains so many ideas for healthy snacks that it would be impossible to list them all here. Some of the best, tastiest and easiest fresh fruit and vegetable snacks include baby carrots or carrot slices, bit size vegetables such as broccoli florets, radishes and green peppers, fresh vegetable and fruit juice and fruit salads.

For a quick and easy fruit salad, try this five minute recipe. Open a can of mandarin oranges and pour it into a bowl, making sure to capture all the delicious juice as well. Cut up a banana, an apple and a nectarine and add them to the bowl. Add some strawberries, blueberries and raisins for extra taste and color, and serve.

Of course fresh fruit also makes a great snack on its own. Snacking on apples, bananas and oranges is a great way to eat healthy and still enjoy delicious snacks. Keeping a bowl of delicious fruit on the table or the coffee table is a great way to encourage the entire family to eat healthier.

The milk and dairy products food group also contains many healthy snack items, including low fat and nonfat yogurt, skim milk, low fat puddings, cheeses and even chocolate milk.

Low fat cuts of prepared meats and low fat varieties of lunch meats make great snacks as well. Sandwiches made with whole grain bread and low calorie spreads like mustard can be a great treat any time of day or night.

Canned tuna (packed in water of course), peanut butter, eggs and egg substitutes, poultry, nuts and beans are also excellent choices for healthy snacks.

When creating healthy snacks, it is important to limit the consumption of high fat foods, and foods high in salt and sodium. Instead of buying snacks in the snack aisle of the grocery store, try making your own using some of the suggestions listed above.

For added variety, try combining several different healthy snacks in unexpected ways. For instance, try spreading peanut butter on pita bread, or use it as a fun dip for apple slices. Or top a whole grain English muffin with tuna and cheese. Place it in the broiler for a few minutes and enjoy a healthy and delicious snack.

Other good ideas for quick and healthy snacks include pairing fresh fruit with nonfat plain or vanilla yogurt, adding fresh fruit slices to cereal, and using fresh fruit and fruit juices to make delicious smoothies.

To perk up bagels that are getting a little stale, try slicing them into thin pieces and arranging them on a baking sheet. Brush them with some low fat salt free butter or margarine, some garlic powder and bake them for 10-12 minutes at 350 degrees. This is a great way to make your own inexpensive and healthy bagel chips without the preservatives or extra sodium found in the store bought variety.

There are of course many other types of healthy snacks, and their variety is only limited by your creativity. It is important to make a variety of healthy snacks, and keep them readily at hand. Replacing all those unhealthy snacks with healthier alternatives is one of the best ways to keep snack cravings from sidetracking your healthy eating goals.

40- Determining if your diet is healthy enough

Everyone wants to eat a healthier diet, but it can sometimes be difficult to know if your diet is healthy enough. There are a number of factors that go into creating a healthy diet, and it is important to evaluate the current state of your diet before embarking on a plan for healthier eating.

There are several questions you should ask yourself when evaluating the healthiness (or lack thereof) of your current eating plan. These questions include:

Do I eat a wide variety of foods?

Variety is one of the most important hallmarks of a healthy diet, since no one food contains all the nutrients needed by the human body. It is important to eat foods from all the major food groups, including grains and breads, fruits and vegetables, milk and dairy products, meats, beans and nuts.

If you find yourself avoiding some food groups, such as vegetables for instance, it may be time to look for a healthier diet.

Do I recognize the importance of cereals, breads and other grain products?

Eating a wide variety of grain based products is important to a healthy diet. Grains and cereals contain a large number of important nutrients, including high levels of dietary fiber.

It is important to choose whole grain products as often as possible, since whole grain products like wheat bread contain more nutrients than more refined white bread and similar products. When eating cereal, it is a good idea to choose whole grain varieties, or those that are enriched with vitamins and minerals.

Do I eat lots of fruits and vegetables?

Many people do not eat sufficient servings of fruits and vegetables every day. Most experts recommend eating between 5 and 9 servings of fruits and vegetables every day, roughly equivalent to 2 cups of fruit and 2 ½ cups of vegetables.

When shopping for vegetables and fruits, it is important to choose a good variety of dark green, dark red, orange and yellow varieties. That is because different colored fruits and vegetables contain a variety of different nutrients, including vitamin C, vitamin A and beta carotene.

Do I eat a good breakfast every morning?

Breakfast, or the absence of it, is often a good indicator of the state of your diet. If you rush out of the house every morning and grab a donut at the local convenience store, chances are your diet can use some work. A healthy breakfast provides a foundation for the rest of the day, helps you avoid cravings and provides much needed nutrition.

Do I choose low fat foods over higher fat alternatives?

This is also an important question to ask yourself. Low fat alternatives are available for a variety of products, including milk, cheese, meats and more.

One part of following a healthy, low fat diet is avoiding prepared foods whenever possible, since prepared foods tend to have higher amounts of fat and sodium than fresh foods.

It is also important to control the amount of fat that is added at the table. Adding things like butter, sour cream and heavy sauces is a sure way to ruin an otherwise healthy meal. Even healthy foods like salads can be sabotaged by the addition of high fat salad dressings. Try using lower fat alternatives like flavored vinegars instead.

Do I drink plenty of water?

Drinking plenty of fresh, pure water is important to maintaining a healthy body and a healthy lifestyle. Water is important to maintaining optimal levels of health.

If you think you need more water, try substituting water for less healthy beverages like soda and coffee.

Am I able to maintain my optimal body weight?

Gaining weight without trying to is often a sign of a poor diet. Following a healthy diet, and getting plenty of regular exercise, is the only way to lose weight and keep it off.

Do I limit the amount of salt, sugar, alcohol and caffeine in my diet?

While all of these elements are fine in moderation, excessive amounts of any of these four can indicate a serious problem with your diet. It is important to limit the amount of unhealthy elements in any diet.

41- Brown bagging it the healthy way

When enjoying a healthy lifestyle, one of the biggest challenges is making meals on the go. Brown bagging is even more difficult when children are involved, but it is still possible to create delicious, nutritious brown bag lunches that the whole family will love.

The most important part of creating healthy, delicious brown bag lunches is choosing the foods that will go into those brown bags. It is important to choose foods that are easy to put together, and to include foods that everyone in the family likes. Including everyone's favorite foods is a great way to make sure the lunches will be eaten instead of traded for Twinkies.

When creating healthy brown bag lunches for yourself and your family, try to choose at least three choices from the following list.

- ➢ At least one fruit or vegetable, either fresh, canned or frozen. Some good choices include apples, bananas and oranges. Fruit salad also makes a great choice for brown bag lunches.

- ➢ A whole grain product like bread, a tortilla shell, a bagel, pasta, rice or muffins.

- ➢ Milk or dairy products like low fat or nonfat yogurt, skim milk, cheese or a yogurt drink or shake.

- ➢ Meat, fish, poultry, eggs, peanut butter, legumes or hummus

- ➢ A healthy vegetable or fruit salad

It is a great idea to involve the whole family in the preparation of these brown bag creations. Why not have a family session where everyone creates their own healthy brown bag lunches using the ingredients you provide? Lay out all the healthy foods, selected from the above list, and let everyone choose their favorites. Involving the kids in meal planning at an early age is a great way to help them learn to make healthy food choices throughout their lives.

Packing those brown bag lunches can be exciting and fun for the whole family. For instance, why not let every member of the family choose his or her own special lunch box or bag? Other good ideas and tips for brown bag lunches include setting aside one shelf in the fridge for lunch fixings and finished lunches, and setting aside a drawer in the cupboard for all the packaging required, such as plastic bags, plastic cutlery, napkins, and straws.

Of course, keeping the variety in brown bag lunches is very important, both for the adults and the kids. There are some great suggestions for keeping everyone from getting bored, including:

> Use a variety of different breads in your sandwiches. Use a combination of wheat bread, rye bread and pumpernickel, in addition to interesting bread alternatives such as tortilla wraps, bread sticks and whole wheat crackers.

> Pack bite size vegetables, such as baby carrots, broccoli florets and pepper slices, along with a low fat dipping sauce.

> Add bit size fruit like grapes, blueberries, orange wedges and strawberries.

> Use only 100% fruit juice in brown bag lunches. Avoid fruit drinks and blends, which often contain less than 10% real fruit.

> Pick up a variety of single serving cereal and let everyone choose their favorites.

> Buy a good selection of flavors of nonfat or low fat yogurt every week, and let everyone choose their favorite flavor every day.

> Pack a variety of dried fruit in your family's brown bag lunches.

Of course the kids are not the only ones who can enjoy healthy brown bag lunches. Mom and dad can also join in the fun. After all, brown bag lunches are a lower cost, and healthier alternative to lunches out.

Some of the most popular choices for brown bag lunches, both for children and their parents, include leftovers from the night before (pasta, rice and potato dishes are great choices), cheese and crackers, leftover veggie pizza, or a quick sandwich rollup using a soft tortilla shell or pita bread.

One great way to enjoy a variety of healthy new foods is to form a lunch partnership with four or five other coworkers. Everyone takes turns bringing lunch for everyone. This can be a great way to enjoy healthy new foods and gather some great new recipes.

42- Planning healthy meals for yourself and your family

Planning healthy meals can be difficult and time consuming, but with some advance planning and some basic knowledge of nutrition, it is easy to create a week's worth of healthy meals that everyone in the family will love.

The key to creating healthy, delicious meals for the family is planning, planning and planning. Planning the week's meals ahead of time is the best way to create meals you can be proud of, while keeping cost and time commitment to a minimum.

Convenience devices such as slow cookers and microwaves can be a huge time saver when planning and preparing meals. There are many delicious and healthy recipes that can be started in the morning and left to cook all day in a crock pot or slow cooker. These are great choices for working families.

In addition, making the meals ahead of time on the weekend and heating them in the microwave is a great way to stretch both your food and your time. There are many microwavable healthy meals you can make at home, and single serving microwave safe containers allow every member of the family to eat on their own schedule.

When planning the meals for the week, it is a good idea to create a chart listing each day's menu and each days' schedule. Planning the quickest, easiest to prepare meals for the busiest days of the week is a smart strategy.

It is a good idea to involve the entire family in creating the week's meal plan. Get everyone's input and note everyone's favorite foods. Of course, that does not mean eating pizza every night or having ice cream for dinner. It is still important to eat healthy meals, and involving your spouse and children in healthy meal planning is a great way to pique their interest in healthy eating at an early age.

It is also a good idea to get the entire family involved in the preparation of the meals. Even children too young to cook can help out by setting out the dishes, chopping vegetables, clearing the table and washing the dishes.

Cooking large quantities of healthy food is a great way to save time. Cooking large amounts of stews, soups, pasta, chili and casseroles can be a huge time saver. Making double and even triple batches of these staple foods, and freezing the leftovers for later use, is a great way to save both time and money.

When freezing leftovers, however, it is important to label the containers carefully, using freezer tape and a permanent marker. Try to keep the oldest foods near the top to avoid having to throw away expired items.

Stocking up on meats when they are on sale is another great way to use that valuable freezer space. Stocking up on such easily frozen foods as chicken, turkey, ground beef, steaks, roasts and chops is a great way to make your food dollar stretch as far as possible while still allowing you and your family to enjoy healthy, delicious meals every day.

Keeping a well stocked pantry is as important as keeping a well stocked freezer. Stocking the pantry with a good supply of staple items like canned vegetables, canned fruits, soup stocks and the like will make healthy meal preparation much faster and easier.

Stocking the pantry can save you money as well as time. Grocery stores are always running sales, and these sales are a great time to stock up. Buying several cases of canned vegetables when they are on sale, for instance can save lots of money and provide the basic ingredients for many nutritious, easy to prepare meals.

Examples of great staples to stock up on include whole grain cereals, pastas, tomato sauce, baked beans, canned salmon, tuna and whole grain breads. It is easy to combine these staples into many great meals on a moment's notice.

43- Getting the most from healthy fruits and vegetables

Fruits and vegetables are among the healthiest of all foods, and the great variety of these foods at the local grocery store makes it easier than every to enjoy great meals and snacks anytime the mood strikes you.

The latest food guidelines recommend that adults eat from five to nine servings of fruits and vegetables every day. While that may seem like a lot, it is an important goal to strive for, and a very reachable one.

A serving of a fruit or vegetable is equal to:

- ➢ 1 medium sized vegetable or fruit (such as an apple, orange or banana)
- ➢ 2 small fruits (such as kiwi fruit or plums)
- ➢ ½ cup of fresh, frozen or canned fruits or vegetables
- ➢ ½ cup of 100% fruit juice
- ➢ ¼ cup of dried fruit
- ➢ 1 cup of green salad

Eating a diet that is rich in fruits and vegetables is a great way to start a healthier lifestyle. Diets high in fruits and vegetables have been shown to reduce the risk of heart disease, diabetes, stroke and even some kinds of cancer. Diets high in fruits and vegetables are also important in maintaining a healthy weight.

Since different varieties of fruits and vegetables contain different types and levels of nutrients, it is important to each a good variety of fruits and vegetables. Eating a good combination of yellow, orange, red and green fruits and vegetables is a great way to ensure adequate levels of nutrition.

Fruits and vegetables are also an important source of fiber. One way to maximize the amount of fiber you get from fruits and vegetables is to eat the entire fruit and vegetable including the edible peel. Eating fruits and vegetables whole, instead of simply drinking fruit juice, is the best way to enjoy the fiber these foods have to offer. Orange juice may be very healthy, but it does not contain the same amount of fiber as a whole orange.

Getting sufficient fiber in the diet offers a great many health benefits, including aiding in digestion, lowering levels of cholesterol in the blood, reducing the risk of heart disease and stroke, and reducing the chances of some forms of cancer. In addition, fiber is though to play an important role in controlling levels of blood sugar in diabetics. Fiber also helps dieters feel full while limiting the number of calories you consume.

Many people wonder if canned and frozen fruits and vegetables are as healthy and nutritious as the fresh varieties. The simple answer to this question is yes. Canned and frozen fruits and vegetables contain just as many vitamins and minerals as their fresh counterparts, so it is fine to replace fresh fruits and vegetables with canned and frozen varieties when fresh ones are not available.

Fresh fruits and vegetables are often less expensive, however, especially when they are in season. In addition, local farmers markets and produce stands are often great sources of the freshest, most delicious fruits and vegetables at some excellent prices.

How vegetables and fruits are prepared is just as important as how they are chosen. It is important to rinse fresh fruit and vegetables thoroughly under clean running water. This step is important in order to remove any dirt, pesticide residue or bacterial contamination. The outermost leaves of lettuce and cabbage should be removed, and the outside of root vegetables like carrots and potatoes should be removed, especially if you plan to consume the skins of those vegetables. Vegetables and fruits should be washed right before they are used in order to keep them as fresh as possible.

The best ways to cook vegetables in order to maintain their freshness are to boil, microwave or steam the veggies until they are tender and crisp. It is best to use as little water as possible when cooking vegetables. That is because overcooking can destroy some of the valuable vitamins and minerals the vegetables contain.

44- Choosing the healthiest frozen meals

When it comes to eating healthy, fresher is almost always better. In some cases, however, it is impossible to cook fresh foods every night. For people on the go, frozen foods can be healthy alternatives to fresh products.

While there is no substitute for a well balanced, fresh cooked meal using plenty of fresh and healthy ingredients, healthy frozen meals can provide a quick and easy alternative for busy people and those who do not have time to cook meals from scratch.

No matter what type of diet you are following, chances are there is a frozen meal available to meet your needs. From low fat to heart healthy to vegetarian meals, there are a great many frozen dinners at the local supermarket or grocery store.

While frozen foods can be very healthy, it is important to keep a close eye out for potentially unhealthy ingredients as you shop. In particular, many frozen and prepared foods have unacceptably high levels of sodium. In addition, many frozen dinners, even those that use the healthiest ingredients, may use preservatives to which some people may be sensitive.

When choosing from among the many brands and varieties of frozen foods on the grocery store shelf, it is important to read the nutritional labels very carefully. These government mandated nutritional labels contain a wealth of information, but it is important to understand how to read them.

Nutritional labels provide information on such imporarnt things as calorie count, number of fat grams and amount of sodium, as well as the percentages of various vitamisn and minerals the food contains.

When examining those nutritional labels, it is important to pay close attention to the portion size. Even a small frozen dinner can be equal to two servings, so if you plan to eat the whole thing yourself, be sure to double the calories, sodium and fat content numbers.

When looking at the amount of fat in a frozen dinner, it is important to follow the widely accepted recommendations to keep the total amount of daily fat to less than 30% of daily calories. Luckily, the new nutritional labels mandated by the government makes this calculation a lot easier. Food manufacturers are required to list the amount of fat their foods contain as a percentage of an average daily diet, so it is easy to tell at a glance if a particular frozen food is a healthy, low fat choice.

In addition to keeping total fat to less than 30% of total calories, it is important to keep saturated fat levels to less than 10% of daily calories. For sodium levels, it is important to limit the amount of sodium to less than 200 milligrams for every 100 calories of food.

In addition, most experts recommend keeping your daily sodium intake to less than 2400 milligrams per day. It is important to read the labels on all frozen foods, even if they are labeled as healthy. While claiming the healthy label obligates food manufacturers to follow certain guidelines, it is still important to review the labels in order to choose the healthiest choices.

When choosing the healthiest meals from among the hundreds of varieties at the average supermarket or grocery store, it is a good idea to choose those that contain at least a half cup of vegetables, fruits or beans. Doing so will help you ensure that the meal you choose is healthy and nutritious.

Finally, since you are in the grocery store already, why not make a stop at the salad bar for a healthy addition to your frozen entrée. Many large grocery store chains have installed wonderful salad bars stocked full of the freshest fruits, vegetables and garnishes, as well as a great selection of low fat and nonfat salad dressings.

45- Creating a healthy fridge

In many ways the refrigerator is the cornerstone of any healthy eating plan. How you stock that fridge can make a huge difference in the success or failure of any healthy eating plan. From what foods it contains, to where they are stored, the refrigerator can be vitally important to healthy eating.

The first step should be to take stock of just what the refrigerator contains. The bachelors among us may already be familiar with this process, but taking stock of the fridge means more than just throwing away those foods that have begun to turn green or grow hair.

Taking stock of the contents of the fridge should mean a monthly review of everything it contains. During this review, separate the healthier foods from the others. It is important to make sure that you have more low fat, high fiber and low sugar foods than high fat low fiber and high sugar ones. If the ratio is off, try to shop for healthier foods.

Another great trick for keeping a healthy refrigerator is to hide the less healthy foods. Try hiding the desserts and other such foods in the crisper, where they will be out of sight and not constantly tempting you. Since fresh fruits and vegetables tend to dry out if they are not used right away, store them in plain sight to increase their likelihood of being eaten. Hiding cakes in the produce drawers, and prominently displaying the fruits and vegetables, is a smart way to keep a healthy fridge.

Another tip is to organize the refrigerator into different sections, and to segregate those sections into sometimes foods (unhealthy choices) and everyday foods (healthy choices). Try to place the healthier foods in the front of the refrigerator, while relegating the unhealthier choices to the back.

Substitution is another great strategy for creating a healthy fridge and a healthy lifestyle. There are low fat and nonfat versions of literally hundreds of different foods. Try substituting skim or 1% milk for whole milk, soft margarines for fattier butter, and low fat sour cream for the full fat varieties. Try replacing fattier meats with leaner ones, or with chicken and fish. Even a simple change, like substituting a soft margarine for butter, can result in significant savings of saturated fat.

For those families with young children, it is important to involve the entire family in healthy eating lifestyles. The habits children learn in childhood often follow them throughout their adult lives, so it makes a lot of sense to get them off to a great start. Try decorating healthy foods with fun stickers, stars, or other colorful items.

Stickers and stars are not the only way to make healthy foods more appealing. Try storing healthy foods with attractive, delicious toppings to make them more interesting and appealing. Try storing a container of berries next to the low fat yogurt, or a bottle of chocolate syrup with the 1% milk. Mixing these foods together is a great way to create healthy snacks quickly.

Another key to creating a healthy refrigerator is to use leftovers wisely. Leftovers can be very useful, and healthy meals make healthy leftovers. Try using leftovers as lunches, or as healthy snacks for the next day.

Ready to eat meals are a great way to encourage healthy eating. Try this handy trick – when you return from your weekly grocery shopping, take the time to create some quick single serving meals and stack them in the fridge. In addition, try making some quick snacks by cutting up fresh fruits and vegetables and storing them in single serving containers.

Using the freezer space in your refrigerator wisely is important as well. Freezing foods that won't be used right away is a great way to make your food dollar go further and to provide quick meals for your family. Try freezing foods in portion sizes. This will make it easier to eat healthier meals, and it will help ensure everyone gets their favorites. When looking at portion sizes, remember that the recommended serving size of meat is 3 ounces, roughly equivalent to the size of a deck of playing cards. The standard serving size for pasta is one cup, while a serving of vegetables is ½ cup.

The freezer can also be a great way to create fun fruit snacks for the

entire family. Freezing healthy fruits like grapes, orange slices and bananas make great snacks for children and adults alike.

46- Making smart food choices with practical foods

Everyone who is trying to follow a healthy eating lifestyle understands the need to buy quality, healthy and practical foods. Practical foods are those foods that are not only healthy but whose benefits extend beyond their mere nutritional value. Such foods are easy to use, and useful in a number of different recipes. Healhty, practical foods, when used on a regular basis, form a great part of a healthy diet, and may even lower the risk of heart disease, cancer and other common illnesses.

One great practical food is the humble tomato. It may not look much like an orange, but the tomato is actually a citrus fruit as well. As such, tomatoes are rich in vitamin C and other antioxidants. In addition, tomatoes are a rich source of lycopene, which has shown promise in preventing certain kinds of cancer.

In addition, tomatoes are easy to use, versatile, and inexpensive. In addition to fresh, in season tomatoes, which are delicious as well as nutritious, tomatoes are available in canned and frozen varieties as well. Tomatoes can be used in so many different ways, and in so many different recipes, that it is always a good idea to have a supply of them on hand in the pantry or the fridge.

Pastas, especially the whole wheat varieties of pastas, are another great example of functional foods. Pastas can also be used in a variety of ways, from simple preparations with simple tomato based sauces, to elaborate creations using shrimp, tuna and other seafood.

Of course, pasta dishes can be healthy or unhealthy, depending on how they are topped. Toppings such as Alfredo sauce or rich cream sauces, should be avoided when trying to follow a healthy diet. As with all foods, such heavy sauces are fine in moderation, but they should not form the bulk of your diet.

Luckily, there are lower fat alternatives to many high fat pasta sauces, and these low fat alternatives should be used whenever possible. Substituting lower fat alternatives for fatty, unhealthy foods is an important skill when it comes to creating a healthy diet.

Whole grain breads, flours and grains are also good examples of hellathy, practical foods. Stocking up on these staples when they are on sale will help ensure that you have everything you need to create the most healthy recipes possible for yourself and your family.

Whole grain products should be substituted for more highly refined breads and cereals whenever possible, since whole grain breads, cereals and grains retain more of their important nutrients than do more highly refined foods.

Starting a healthy eating program using practical foods is easy. Start by taking a personal inventory of your current diet, including where it is good and where it can use some improvement. Learn to assess the personal health risks created by your current diet (your family physician can be of particular help here). A physician or dietitian can be a big help in putting together a list of healthy, easy to use, practical foods you can use to change your diet for the better.

It is also a good idea to use your interest in healthy eating to create and use exciting new recipes. There are a great many healthy eating recipes available, both on the internet and in cookbooks. Seek out some of these recipes and try using your favorite healthy staples to create some wonderful dishes.

For some ideas on how to use practical foods morning, noon and night, try some of these great ideas:

Breakfast:

- ✓ Include some healthy staples, and some healthy fruits in your breakfast. For instance, pair healthy oatmeal with blueberries, or whole wheat or wheat bran cereal with strawberries or bananas.
- ✓ Try mixing a healthy cereal like All Bran into your nonfat or low fat yogurt. It will perk up your plain yogurt and give it a great crunch.

✓ Fresh fruit is also a great addition to yogurt. Try buying plain, nonfat yogurt and mixing in your own raspberries, blueberries and strawberries. You will save money and enjoy a healthy breakfast.

✓ Instead of high fat butter, spread your toast with apple butter or soy nut butter instead. Always try to use whole grain varieties of bread like wheat or rye.

✓ Drink a glass of 100% fruit juice with breakfast every day. Orange juice, grape juice, apple juice and grapefruit juice are all great choices.

✓ Blend 1% milk or soy milk with fresh pineapple for a healhy, delicious breakfast smoothie. These smoothies are great for people on the go.

Lunch and dinner ideas

✓ Make a great tuna salad with grated carrots, green peppers, red peppers, garlic and onion.

✓ Make a dish of fresh whole grain pasta and top it will homemade tomato sauce and fresh home grown herbs.

✓ Use healthy foods like onions and leeks, along with tomatoes, as a great side dish.

✓ Grill healthy fish and serve with a healthy side salad.

✓ Try some low fat soups like spinach and broccoli soup.

✓ Make a great vegetable stir fry with olive oil.

Healthy snacks

Of course no plan for healthy eating is complete without some great healthy snacks. Below are some of our favorite healthy snacks for those on the go.

✓ A piece of fresh fruit, like an apple, orange or banana, always makes a great snack. Keep a bowl of fruit on your kitchen counter for easy access.

✓ Try mixing nuts and dried fruit for a great homemade trail mix. Hikers and non hikers alike will enjoy this healthy snack.

✓ Treat yourself to a great glass of orange, tomato or cranberry juice before you leave the house in the morning.

✓ Keep a supply of broccoli florets, baby carrots and other bite size vegetables, and some healthy dip, on hand.

✓ Make your own fruit salad with oranges, bananas, raspberries, blueberries, strawberries and other favorites.

47- Buying healthy foods at the grocery store

The local grocery store is a great place to find healthy, nutritious foods. Unfortunately, it is also a place to find less healthy foods and many junk foods. Learning how to follow a healthy lifestyle means learning how to shop for the healthiest foods, and learning how to avoid temptation.

Learning to read labels is an important skill for any healthy shopper. The information on nutritional labels is very valuable, providing complete information on the percentage of many vitamins and minerals a particular food contains. In addition, nutritional information labels provide valuable information on things like the amount of calories, number of at grams, percentage of total fat and amount of fiber each food contains. It is important to choose those foods that have the best nutritional qualities as you roam the local grocery store.

There are some important guidelines to follow to make sure that every trip to the grocery store will be a healthy experience. After all, you cannot have a healthy refrigerator or a healthy dinner table without first stocking your kitchen pantry with the healthiest foods available.

One of the best pieces of advice is probably something you have heard a million times, and that is to never go grocery shopping when you are hungry. Even if it means stopping for a quick snack on your way, it is important to not enter the supermarket while you are hungry. Hungry shoppers make bad choices, and those unhealthy choices will be around long after your hunger has abated.

Another good trick is to hit the produce section of your grocery store first. Fill up your food basket with healthy, nutritious fruits and vegetables. Not only will this allow you to stock the fridge and the pantry with healthy choices, but it will leave less room for all those less healthy foods.

It is also important to always make a detailed shopping list before hitting the grocery store. A well thought out grocery list keeps you from overspending, and also helps keep you from succumbing to the temptation of less healthy junk foods. To keep a detailed list of what you need on your next shopping list, try keeping a notepad by the fridge or on the dining room table. Write down each item as you think of it, and come shopping day, you will have a complete list of everything you need to buy.

As you shop around the grocery store, it is a good idea to take advantage of the many low fat foods that fill grocery store shelves. There are low at varieties of many foods, including milk and dairy products, meats and cheeses, even cakes and pies. Most of these products contain all the taste of the full fat products, without all the fat.

When shopping for low fat foods, however, be on the lookout for extra sugar content. This is not so much a concern with milk and dairy products, but it is sometimes a concern with low fat baked goods. Some manufacturers pack their low fat baked goods with extra sugar, so it pays to be a smart label reader.

As long as you watch sugar content, however, low fat desserts and sweets are excellent choices. When grocery shopping, try to choose naturally lower fat alternatives, such as angel food cake, fig bars and vanilla wafers. Buying smaller portion sizes is another smart strategy for enjoying sweets while limiting fat and calories.

Another smart strategy is to choose whole grain breads and cereals whenever possible. Whole grains contain more fiber and other nutrients than do more processed foods, so buying whole grains makes a lot of sense.

When shopping for the healthiest cereals in the grocery store, it is helpful to understand how the cereal aisle of the typical grocery store is arranged. Shelf space at a grocery store is in high demand and short supply, and cereal manufacturers take advantages of this fact in their store shelf marketing. In general, the less healthy, sugar laden cereals are arranged at kid height, while the more adult, healthier products are on the top shelves.

That is one reason why your kids are always trying to put those sugar cubes disguised as cereal in your cart as you shop. Choosing the healthier cereals from the top shelves is a good strategy, but it is still important to read the labels to make sure you are getting what you think you are.

ABOUT THE AUTHOR

Al Fiqi Haytham is a Cairo born criminal lawyer who obtained his Bachelor's Degree in Law from the University of Mansoura in 1997. His is a correspondent and editor for the New Egypt press and is supported by the Supreme Council of the Press. He has also published various legal essays and has acted as an adviser to nursing staff in many different medical facilities.

In his free time, Al Fiqi Haytham enjoys Play chess ,Playing pool ,Read the legal and scientific books ,Shopping ,Watch foreign movies ,Listening to Beethoven pieces ,Driving.You can reach him via his blog (http://haythamalfiqi.blogspot.com/) or via email (haythamalfiqi0@gmail.com) to get information about new releases.